I CAN SIT AGAIN

I CAN SIT AGAIN

Non-Surgical Treatment
for Tailbone Pain

Dr. Jennifer K. Stebbing, DO

NEW YORK

LONDON • NASHVILLE • MELBOURNE • VANCOUVER

I Can Sit Again

Non-Surgical Treatment for Tailbone Pain

Published in New York, New York, by Morgan James Publishing in partnership with Difference Press. Morgan James is a trademark of Morgan James, LLC.
www.MorganJamesPublishing.com

ISBN 9781642799101 paperback
ISBN 9781642799118 eBook
ISBN 9781642799125 audiobook
Library of Congress Control Number: 2019919224

Cover Design Concept:
Jennifer Stimson

Cover Design by:
Megan Dillon
megan@creativeninjadesigns.com

Interior Design by:
Christopher Kirk
www.GFSstudio.com

Cover Design Concept:
Bethany Davis

Cover Design Concept:
The Author Incubator

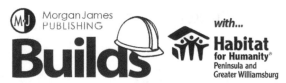

Morgan James is a proud partner of Habitat for Humanity Peninsula and Greater Williamsburg. Partners in building since 2006.

Get involved today! Visit
MorganJamesPublishing.com/giving-back

Thank you to my patients and friends in New Hampshire who have supported me, challenged me, and helped me grow professionally.

Thank you to three of the important men in my life:

For my son, Julian, who has been a steady companion through my process of redefining my professional life. There is nothing more grounding then having to look into the mirror and face what may not be an ideal habit. Being your mother has been the biggest blessing and challenge. Thank you. I love you.

To "Uncle" Dr. Patrick Clary, my hospice and palliative care mentor, colleague, and friend. I learned to love medicine again as I learned the value of having clear, defined emotional boundaries between what is mine and what is someone else's suffering.

To Dr. Jonathon Fenton, DO, whose collegial generosity towards teaching me has not only elevated my confidence but changed my philosophy of practice from one of apprehension to one of abundance. There is no shortage of people with chronic pain or arthritis that need to be treated with regenerative orthopedic medicine. There is a shortage of physicians that need to be trained. I hope to follow in your footsteps, fostering and elevating the next generation of physicians.

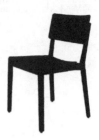

TABLE OF CONTENTS

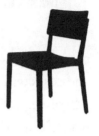

Chapter 1

I CAN'T SIT. WHAT DO I DO?

"I've fallen. I landed hard right on my tailbone area, and I've not been the same since."

This is not an uncommon story that women have come into my office with, but there are variations. "I delivered my baby, he was big, I tore, and I've had pain in my tailbone since." Or "I was playing a sport, I jumped up and landed on one leg, and I've had discomfort in my bum since." Or "I was in a car accident, I stomped on my brake to avoid the impact, and I have back problems with pain that goes into my derriere." In another situation, someone had an injury with a large scar that caused pain in this same area.

Every one of these situations had pain that interfered with sitting. Sitting is an integral part of everyone's life. Sitting allows you to drive a car, eat meals, and rest comfortably on the sofa at the end of the day. Effectively, it allows you to be a social individual. You sit with your family during mealtimes. A date to the movies is enjoyable as you settle comfortably into your seat. Eating out or having a cup of coffee or tea with friends usually involves sitting. Work or school requires that you sit. When your ability to sit is affected, the rest of your life is compromised as a consequence.

Chronic pain interferes with your ability to think. It affects your ability to find pleasure in life, as the pain is not distractible. This can lead to depression. It leads to compensatory or altered movement patterns that may cause other problems. For instance, some people find that if they cross one leg over the other and get the weight off the side that has pain, they can sit for longer, but the issue starts to involve the lower back, the neck, or the shoulders, as the alignment becomes twisted. One thing leads to another. Sometimes the pain causes you to yell at the people you most care about like your kids or your spouse. It causes you to feel irritable, then the guilt sets in. You judge yourself and your ability to parent or be a good partner. Your sense of who you are starts to be lost.

Tailbone pain, as some people call it, may be exactly what the issue is. Alternatively, the pain may actually be a sacroiliac joint issue, or nerve, fascia, or muscle pain. This is a complex area. It is difficult to diagnose. X-rays or MRIs don't always help with figuring out the pain. One doctor may offer a solution that is very different than another doctor. This can be very confusing. I'm sure that you just want a diagnosis or a reasonable explanation of what is causing your pain and all your options for treating it. I always tell people that just because a doctor doesn't understand your pain doesn't mean it doesn't exist. Osteopathic or chiropractic treatment offers a respite or relief of pain for a short period. This starts to give you hope that there is something that can be done about your pain. Physical therapy can also be beneficial. You do the exercises as you were told to, with improvement but not complete relief. Acupuncture may work wonders, or it may not work at all. You've changed your diet. You've done cleanses. You try to reduce the stress in your life, but it's difficult if you are the prime wage-maker or carry the insurance for the family.

Your biggest fear is that it won't go away, that you will miss out on your children's activities, that your employment is in jeopardy, that you are not worthy of feeling whole again. Sometimes it is easier to deal with the pain or discomfort that you have rather than risk it getting worse. Your ability to make clear, thoughtful decisions becomes clouded by the pain and lack of sleep.

However, there are treatment options for all these situations. My practice is geared toward treating pain that prevents you from participating in life fully. I have helped many people with various reasons for not being able to sit comfortably. Your pain is real, even if no one else has figured out why. In this book, I will discuss these non-surgical treatment options that are medically sound and have been proven clinically for decades. I have many tools in my bag to do this with the end goal of getting you sitting comfortably again.

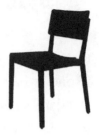

Chapter 2

IS MY PAIN REAL?

P ain was not something that my medical education taught me about. It wasn't until I started my training as a hospice and palliative care physician that I was exposed to how to quantify pain. We asked patients to rate their pain on a scale from zero to ten, where five is a level of pain where one would find the pain an interference to a phone conversation and need to get off. This level of pain is not distractible. I had experienced ankle sprains in high school but nothing above the level of a four out of ten. As I saw patients near their end of life, I was taught that the brain perceives all pain in the same area of the brain. Pain can be physical pain, emotional pain, and/or spiritual pain. Our brain experiences this pain the same. This means that it's hard to figure out where the pain originates if one is only spending fifteen minutes or less, the standard length of time in the conventional medical model, with a patient. I realized this as I pursued my sports medicine training. Treatment of solely physical pain without considering other potential causes of pain (emotional and spiritual), may not be possible. I have noticed this especially after a patient has had a few surgical operations that have not addressed their pain. Now their pain is more complicated. It is not just physical; there is also some emotional scarring, perhaps even PTSD, that needs to be treated at the same time.

My hospice training taught me about pain, however there is nothing like experiencing pain. There are two examples in my life where I experienced pain that I would rate as eight out of ten on the pain scale. On one occasion, I had no physical trauma. I developed severe unrelenting back pain two days after the Boston Marathon bombings in 2013. I was examined osteopathically and there was no alignment issue. One of my colleagues suggested that perhaps I had depleted my fight or flight hormones, epinephrine (adrenaline) and norepinephrine (noradrenaline) during the intense stress of that day. I took a supplement for about a month and my back pain resolved on its own. In this situation, none of the treatment options that I mention in this book would have worked. However, given my experience, I would recognize this emotional trauma that manifested physically and offer options for treatment. The second example occurred nine months after my child was born. The pain that I experienced was exhausting. It wasn't something that I would wish upon anyone, but I believe that my experience with pain happened so that I could better relate to my patients. I believe that I am guided by what happens to me. It's my choice to decide how to react to a situation; however, there is always something to be learned or gleaned from an experience that I can pass on to others.

Let me tell you in more detail about my second experience with pain. I really wanted to be a mother. I was not married and therefore pursued in vitro with sperm donation as a way to get pregnant and experience all the joys and struggles of being a mother. I followed all the doctor's recommendations without being worried or fearful of anything. I expectcd to get pregnant despite my advanced age of thirty-seven years old, and if not, I was going to adopt. I got pregnant and delivered my son vaginally, which was important to me, as I knew I would not have help in the weeks that followed delivery.

As any parent knows, until the child sleeps through the night, you don't either. Initially, the daily tiredness was not an issue, but once I started working, it was much more apparent. When my son was nine months old, I fell asleep with him in the crook of my right arm after nursing at night. When I awoke, one of my ribs near my sternum had moved out of place. My ligaments were still relaxed by the pregnancy hormones, allowing the rib-sternum joint to be more mobile than normal. The traction of my son's body weight on my arm caused a force to be generated in this area which my body could not hold. I had pain over my sternum. It was visibly swollen. It hurt to breathe. In my exhausted state, it took a while to figure out what to do next. I sought the care of an osteopathic colleague. The osteopathic treatment did not change the pain, which started to involve my shoulder. It hurt to move my shoulder, and I started to develop a frozen shoulder. It was impossible to not move it as a single parent trying to lug around a cumbersome car seat or hold a growing boy. Nursing was excruciating. And it was at night that the pain escalated. I didn't sleep. I was grouchy. I was short with people. I did not feel like socializing. I was irritable, almost angry, all the time. I could not think straight. I finally decided to pursue physical therapy and massage therapy. They kept all the motion in my arm. The pain was high with these treatments. I did not want to get a steroid shot, one of my other options, because I was nursing. Finally, after a few months, I decided to treat the original injury with prolotherapy, a injection-based treatment that I use with my patients all the time to great effect.

Prolotherapy is the original modern-day regenerative treatment. *Prolo-* comes from the word "proliferate," which suggests growth. It consists of injections into the area that is injured. I was scared to have the injections done. I was scared that my pain would escalate. I knew there was no surgical treatment. Because I had not experienced the benefit of being treated with prolotherapy, although I was seeing the benefit in patients that I treated, I was not totally convinced that it would work. Prolotherapy involves using a small gauge needle to inject onto bone. Preforming it on myself was more complicated- I had to guide it by looking backwards in the mirror while being careful to avoid my lungs when I injected my ribs and sternum. My healing started then.

After I treated myself, the pain started to change in this area. My practice of medicine also changed. I started to do more prolotherapy, becoming more proficient with my needle placement and confident about the benefits, but my shoulder was still an issue. I couldn't treat my right shoulder with my dominant right hand and there were no other physicians in the area that practiced prolotherapy. Typically, frozen shoulder pain lasts about six months if not treated because the pain encourages you not to move your arm and you are left with a shoulder that does not move fully. The range of motion is compromised. I instinctively knew that I needed to keep my shoulder moving despite the pain.

As fall approached, a number of my colleagues were gathering in Madison, Wisconsin for a conference. I had met these colleagues in Honduras at a two-week Hackett Hemwell medical mission, where I was taught how to treat patients with prolotherapy. During this conference, my shoulder was injected by a colleague. It was the first time I had pain relief in months. Once I had relief from pain, it opened my professional world. I wanted to help people to experience the benefits of prolotherapy even more than I had before. Only a few injections had been needed to move my pain from a level of five or six out of ten to nearly zero. It was miraculous. Over the years since then, I have had some wonderful success stories treating people with injection therapies. I'd like to share two of these stories with you.

Ted was a runner who had recurring back pain. The pain began to escalate. He described being treated by a chiropractor over the years, which was extremely beneficial. However, more recently, he was not holding the adjustments. As an osteopath, I have treated low back pain by relaxing the psoas muscle or aligning the spine. This situation mimicked situations that I too had experienced. When spinal alignment adjustment is needed over and over again, the issue is that the ligaments are weakened. When the ligaments are weakened, the muscles nearby tighten to hold the joints in place. Sometimes some of the muscles are tighter than others, pulling the joints out of alignment. Muscle spasms can cause back pain. In Ted's situation, I initially treated the muscle spasms with dry needling the trigger points. This involved using an acupuncture needle to release the muscle spasms. I did this with the use of ultrasound, which allowed me to visualize the needle. The goal with this treatment session was to reduce Ted's overall pain.

Then, I treated the ligaments in his low back and pelvis. The cluneal nerves that were also involved in the pain that he experienced in his lower back and occasionally in his tailbone/sacral area were also treated. The treatment that I used included prolotherapy, trigger point release, nerve hydro-dissection, and osteopathic manipulation. These will all be described later. This was a comprehensive treatment session not, as the insurance would like to dictate, a separate visit for each of the different procedures that were done. It took two treatment sessions to remove the everyday, low-level pain that he experienced, and it took another three to four treatment sessions to stabilize the ligaments. He is now running again and has not experienced a recurrence of his back pain.

Another example is Joy, who I treated after she had an accident where surgery was needed to correct a complex fracture. Although this example is specific, regenerative orthopedic medicine still plays an important role after surgery where there continues to be pain. Joy came to my office a year after a ski accident where she suffered a tibial plateau fracture and dislocation of her knee. She had already had six surgeries and still had pain, a lot of scar tissue, and was contemplating an amputation of her joint. She came to me for a second opinion after a surgeon recommended another surgery to remove the scar tissue. She was limited in motion and could not walk without assistive devices. What was most astounding to me was the nature of the tissue around all the scar tissue. It was shiny, rosy, and tight from the underlying swelling in the tissue. It was sensitive to light touch. There was no hair growth to her lower leg compared to the other side. The skin was warmer to the touch than the other side. The pain that she was experiencing was certainly coming from the scar, and I quickly recognized it as RSD (reflex sympathetic dystrophy, now known as complex regional pain syndrome), something I learned in medical school but had never seen in practice. RSD is caused by an injury to the nerves. During Joy's multiple surgeries, the scars had severed a number of the nerves that gave sensation to her skin. As the nerves started to grow back, they could not grow through the scar. They became swollen and started to cause her debilitating pain.

We talked about the treatments that would be necessary, and I was honest about not knowing exactly where this would take us. The injury and the consequential surgeries, some of which were absolutely necessary, created a complex puzzle where the treatment would guide the next treatment. I was absolutely certain that Joy should not amputate her leg. She was extremely proactive, researching many options for treatment, always coming back to me for the discussion. We treated the scars, the knee joint, the supportive tissues (nerve, fascia, ligaments, and capsule around the knee), and recognized that she had also injured her ankle in the same accident and treated both the ankle and the fibula at the knee as well. Initially, I treated Joy with prolotherapy, but we rapidly added platelet-rich plasma (PRP), to encourage healing more rapidly. I had to take more blood and process it sterilely to ensure we had enough volume to treat everything. She took the recommended supplements, and we used a knee brace to assist during healing. She saw a number of other people for areas that they specialized in—massage, physical therapy, acupuncture etc. She saw two other colleagues of mine to help assist in decision-making. She had another arthroscopic surgery to better evaluate the inside of her joint and received bone marrow derived stem cells.

Joy continues to communicate with me, although I moved from the area. She can now walk without a limp. She can hike, and she is active again. Most importantly, she did not pursue amputation in a desperate attempt to get out of pain. I gave her hope and helped provide the framework and much of the treatment to start her healing. However, it was her persistence and ownership of being the master of her own domain that allowed it to happen. She invested in herself. I love her as a friend. For me, it is not possible to do this type of work and not develop a bond with the person that I am treating.

I can treat pain because I understand pain. I understand the depression that occurs when you can't move, sit, reach, or walk comfortably. I understand how hard it is to make decisions when your body is exhausted. I understand the apprehension in making decisions because you don't have all the information. I want to restore your hope that there are solutions to getting treated.

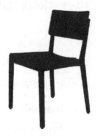

Chapter 3

WHAT ARE SOME TREATMENT OPTIONS?

T he sacral discomfort that you have is treatable. In this chapter, I will discuss the treatment options that I provide and review a few important concepts. In subsequent chapters, I'll dive into these treatment options more deeply.

In general, I use injections to treat you. Although I will concentrate on teaching you about the injections that I do, my other passion is using my hands to treat osteopathically. I love to work with people's bodies to gently lengthen the tissues and correct muscle tension. The combination of both types of treatment I describe as the yin and yang. The injections can cause pain. Your sympathetic, or fight or flight, nervous system can get wired during these treatments while the osteopathic treatments will calm you, activating your parasympathetic nervous system. Even light touch from a skilled practitioner can be beneficial to the healing process.

An important concept to understand is that this treatment is a process. Unless you had a very specific accident, like Joy did, most pain develops over time. One injury has a compounding effect on another. As was the case with both Joy and Ted, the injection treatments occurred over a period of months, and although I offered the two of them similar treatments, the way they were done and what was injected varied. I want you to know that there is no specific treatment algorithm. The way that you are treated will not be exactly the same as someone else and will need to be adjusted as you heal. I love the concept of treating the individual versus treating the masses.

I divide the treatments that I offer into three tiers. Which of these tiers will benefit you will depend on how much pain you have, the degree of your injury, and how quickly you want to be treated. I will discuss each of these tiers in more detail in future chapters.

The first tier is the age-proven treatment called prolotherapy. It uses dextrose, sugar water, as the substance that is injected. The first time I ever heard about prolotherapy, I didn't understand the concept, which I will discuss in much more detail in Chapter 6. Like most doctors, I couldn't get past "sugar water." Since then, I've seen the benefit of prolotherapy in myself and many patients that I have treated. I've effectively proven its benefit to myself.

In the second tier, called platelet-rich plasma (PRP), I use platelets found in your bloodstream. These are injected into the injured area creating a much stronger healing response than prolotherapy.

Stem cells are the third tier. This tier is reserved for more severe injuries or arthritis after the soft tissue structures have been treated.

New options for treatment are always being developed. Knowing when to use what treatment and what patients are appropriate for each treatment is my role as a physician. I continually learn and incorporate new technology. That being said, I am not currently using stem cells that are acquired from other humans. I want to make sure that they have a proven safety record.

There are a few other tools in my toolbox. In Ted's case, I mentioned trigger point release. Trigger points are a localized muscle spasm that develop as a secondary issue. For example, a trigger point can develop because you lengthened a muscle too fast, as is the case in someone who runs quickly to get out of traffic and develops a calf spasm. It can develop when a muscle is totally fatigued, as in the case of marathon runners whose bodies have been depleted of all sources of fuel. But most commonly, trigger points develop when the ligaments that hold a joint in place are stretched out or loosened. The muscles that help move the joint tense up to support it. This happens regularly in people with all the reasons for tailbone pain. I will go into more details about this in Chapter 6.

Perineural treatment and its more elaborate version, nerve hydro-dissection treatment, provide another avenue to treat pain that is nerve related. The sensory nerves provide feeling to the skin. When they are damaged by a scar, as was Joy's case, they start to talk. One nerve starts to talk to another nerve. The musical term "cacophony" comes to my mind. The big picture is that the nerves aren't happy, and the desperation that you may feel may be as dramatic as Joy's desire to amputate her leg. In both of these treatments, sugar water is used to bathe the nerve. Perineural treatment occurs with shallow injections under the skin along the nerve pathway. Hydro-dissection treatment involves looking at the nerve with ultrasound, finding where it is compressed within the tissue, and using a jet of this same sugar water to open up or unzip the fascia that is squeezing the nerve, which causes the problem.

There are other ways that other physicians and non-physicians alike may treat your tailbone pain. In general, it is important to have a team that includes at a minimum a physical therapist. These people help augment your healing. Other members of the team can include those who do body work, such as osteopaths, chiropractors, and massage therapists. Your other doctors, acupuncturists, exercise specialists, mental health providers, and nutritionists are also vital members of your team. I especially like to have someone trained in functional medicine, Ayurvedic medicine, or naturopathic medicine involved.

The success that you have with treatment is partially dependent on getting the right diagnosis, a comprehensive treatment plan, and correct placement of the injected ingredient. However, I also need your help along the way. There are things that you can do to participate in healing. This is the hard work. My job, comparably, is easy. Since your body is innately trying to heal and repair itself all the time, I'd love for you to address your bad habits. Healing is slowed down by nicotine in whatever form it is taken. Many people, when they drink, smoke. Others just drink. The alcohol that you consume provides only empty calories. Alcohol has a profoundly negative effect on your health over time. There was one study that showed that it lowers your body's innate circulating stem cell levels. If you can't stop by yourself, ask for help. Alcoholism is a disease. It's really hard to be a restrained alcoholic without slowly falling into the need to use more over time. Twelve-step programs have been phenomenally supportive and beneficial and are located in every town in this nation. Asking for help is a sign of bravery and likely will help to increase your success.

When the repair process is greater than cells can handle, they become damaged, the DNA can be changed, and disease occurs. Food is medicine. What you choose to put into your body assists with the reparative processes that occur daily and removes some toxic exposure to pesticides, herbicides, and other chemicals added to processed foods that are not beneficial to our bodies. There are experts who can help with identifying food allergies and treating injury to the intestinal wall that prevent absorption of the proper nutrients. Most Americans are sick in various degrees. Obesity is the most obvious marker of this, even if there are no other issues. This is the time to care of yourself. For most people, regardless of their diet, the right supplements from the right company can make a difference. Drinking half your body weight in ounces of water per day is a great goal, unless you have congestive heart failure and/or a fluid balance issue. Movement every day and every hour during the day is vitally important to maintaining health. Sitting is not your long-term friend. Exercise plays a part in this; in fact, there are communities where walking everywhere has shown to be beneficial. I will more thoroughly discuss ways that you can help heal yourself in Chapter 7.

Finding the joy within you occurs as you reflect on your own self. Trying to get rid of your own habitual thought processes, such as self-judging, can be a life-long endeavor. When this occurs, however, there is a lot of room for love. These same issues will be reiterated in this book and, if we meet, will come up again. This work that you do is vitally important for your own health. The more you invest in your own health, the better you will feel and the better the outcome of any treatment.

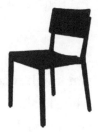

Chapter 4

HOW DO I DECIDE WHAT TO DO?

In the beginning, anyone that gets injured hopes that the injury will heal on its own. There is an expectation that this will happen because it did when we were kids. Granted, time has passed, and we know we don't heal as quickly, but the expectation still exists that we will heal. We *should* heal. So when the days go by and suddenly you realize that the issue that you had last March when you slipped in the parking lot at the ski hill and landed flat on your rear still exists, should you wait another week? There is a part of your brain that recognizes that this is outside of normal and perhaps there is something more you can do, but the other part of your brain that knows that you should and can heal is overpowering it. This is normal behavior; it's new to be injured. The issue then becomes that pain is normal. A certain amount of discomfort is expected while healing, but as the weeks go by, this becomes the new normal.

In the beginning, if the pain is not distractible, it is not an emergency to get it fixed. There are other things, like trying to get the kids to their after-school activities and finding childcare when work engagements arise that need to be attended to first. So the logical choice for that brain of yours that expects you to get better is to do nothing. It's an option and one that most people take. We were taught to press on in high school sports. "No pain, no gain" was the football team's motto. Commercials on TV suggest that this should be done as well.

The next normal sequence of events that occur after an injury, whether it is what seemed to be a minor fall that knocked the wind out of you or a more serious whiplash injury, would be to talk to your friends about their experiences with pain. Usually they have some suggestions for what worked for them. Word of mouth is a powerful marketing tool, no doubt. Massage therapists, chiropractors, and physical therapists all are great next steps. Many times, they have seen the injury before and can recognize what is expected behavior for an injury while healing or what is outside normal healing. This is what separates the good from

the great in any specialty in medicine. Massage therapists can feel the difference from one week to the next
and can tell that the tissue relaxes while it heals. Many
are intuitive, reading energy or using other senses to
gauge what is going on. When the injury is stuck in
its healing and keeps winding back up, they recognize
that there is more going on and can encourage you to
get more advice.

Likewise, chiropractors may find that they have
to continually realign your leg length or readjust your
pelvis because the ligaments are not holding the bony
structure in place. Some great chiropractors can assess
muscle tension and will vary their techniques, adjust-
ing for what they feel. They recognize reoccurring
patterns that aren't getting better, and when they do,
they are curious enough to acknowledge that what
they are doing may not be enough for the patient.
These chiropractors are truly some of your closest
allies. They have your best interest in mind. They may
refer you to physical therapy. Physical therapists have
such a diverse background in training. They specialize according to what their interests are and can dive
deep into one type of treatment regimen that they use
in multiple areas of the body. As their career goes on,
they acquire a number of treatment regimens that they
become really skilled at and can individualize treatment for each patient. Typically, it is the physical

therapist that recognizes abnormal patterns that may require a physician.

Orthopedic surgeons provide the front line for evaluating injuries and arthritis in today's world. Their expertise lies in fracture care and surgical treatment options. I value their skills in advanced arthritis and fractures, however there are physicians, like me, that are trained in non-surgical treatment options. This is a better option for you. The treatment options in the "gray area," as I call it, are non-surgical and proactive, allowing you to postpone or even avoid surgery. It's easy to get lost in the system and not get your problem addressed, if you go the wrong doctor. Your pain is real, and it is probably not being caused by a fractured tailbone, and even if it is, the likelihood of doing surgery for this reason is really low.

I provide care to patients in the gray area! I am personally a sports medicine physician trained in the sub-specialty field of regenerative orthopedics. Physicians who sub-specialize in regenerative orthopedics all take courses and further their education after doing a three- or four-year residency and sometimes an extra year, called a fellowship year. By definition, the training involves extensive anatomy knowledge, ultrasound training, reading of x-rays and MRIs, and proficient use of needles and anesthesia, as well as recognizing who needs surgery. During the course of my training,

I have seen the results of human error in diagnosis and treatment. I have malpractice coverage because things can and do go wrong. I know that infections can be caused by injection techniques, and I take extra steps to avoid infections and any injury from treatment. For me, this specialization took an additional eight years of training after college. However, the years after training provided for the acquisition of wisdom and experience. This is what you want when your pain does not go away.

Pat was in her eighties when she showed up in my office. She was a spry, very educated retired professor. Her initial complaint was thigh pain to the outside of her thigh. This required that she sit or use a walker to get around. It affected every waking moment of her day. What happened to the golden years, she wondered? On exam, she had extreme weakness of her glute muscles. There were trigger points, which I initially treated with osteopathic manipulation and dry needling. This removed her pain in her legs for a few days, which allowed her to gain confidence in the process. But the pain returned. Over the course of a few months, I treated her with a combination of prolotherapy, nerve hydro-dissection, trigger point release, and later platelet-rich plasma. Once her pain was removed, she benefited from physical therapy, initially starting in a pool, and then progressed with body weight, bands, balance, and strength-based exercises. She took my recommendations to heart, actively making a conscious decision to stay out of pain. She is aware that she needs to move every day. This has given her back her life. She no longer needs a walker.

"You've given me hope," people say to me with tears in their eyes, frequently. I understand the grief of losing your identity as an athlete when you fall and can't perform physically. I understand the difficulty of making decisions when you are not sleeping because of pain. I understand the shaming that occurs with other medical professionals who work in the black and white zone and tell you that your pain is in your head or that you will have to live with it as there is nothing that can be done. There are a number of options that can be used to treat your pain, but first I need to determine what the problem is. In the next chapter, I will discuss what occurs in the initial visit with me. Your job as your read through the remaining chapters is to decide whether you want to "let it burn," "dim the lights," or "put out the fire."

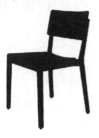

Chapter 5

WHAT DO I NEED TO TELL MY DOCTOR?

"I'm so happy to meet you," I'll say the first time we meet. By the end of the appointment, I hope you feel the same. In this chapter, I will discuss what happens during the appointment and why the information that you tell me is important. The appointment is divided into three different steps: the interview (during which we review tests and lab results if you have them), a thorough evaluation, and finally a review of the recommendations.

The interview is the most important aspect to the visit. It's the time when you get to know me, and I get to know you. You've done this before in other doctor's offices; usually though, you are trying to get everything you need to say out quickly. During our visit, which can last anywhere between forty-five to ninety minutes, you get my undivided attention. I want to know about all the different injuries in your life. The ankle sprains, car accidents, and abuse can have a bearing on what you describe as your tailbone pain. This is not a time to be discriminatory and hold back information because you don't think it is necessary. The whole body is so interconnected that I want to know the big picture of what it has experienced.

Sandra was a patient of mine who had pain or discomfort in many different areas. She was a professor and very capable of defining what type of discomfort or pain she had. She was hypermobile, meaning that she had greater than the normal amount of movement in her joints. Her pain was widespread; it was achy, constant, and interfered with sleep. It increased with any kind of activity. She was afraid of hurting herself by doing too much. One day she came in with sharpie-painted Xs in all the areas that bothered her that week. The pattern started to link together. I recognized that it wasn't her joints that were injured, but rather the muscular and fascia attachments between her pelvis, ribs, and shoulder blade. I treated her at the Xs with prolotherapy and she did really well, returning to her goal of running. I guided the treatment with the knowledge that she was hypermobile and the visual clues that all the Xs gave me.

There are other aspects to the interview. I want to know all the surgeries and other medical issues in your history. The surgeries are injuries. They leave scars. The incisions that are made at the time of surgery can cut sensory nerves. These nerves give feeling to the skin, but are also important to the tissue below them, providing them with nutrition and a sense of health. When these nerves are injured, the tissue beneath them may be more vulnerable to injury and have a harder time healing. The other amazing thing that happens in our bodies is that, in an attempt to heal, they will try to grow the nerves back together. We know that nerves can grow back about a centimeter a year. The issue with scars is that nerves can get stuck in the scar and start to ball up on themselves as they grow and create a scar neuroma. Scar neuromas cause pain. Usually the scar is tender to the touch or has red blotches or a difference of color or there is localized swelling in the area.

Lisa was sixty-two when she came in for an evaluation of her knee. She had recently had arthroscopic knee surgery to trim her meniscus. She had improved for a few weeks after the surgery, and then she started to experience pain. Six weeks after the surgery, her pain escalated. She could barely walk. Her x-ray was not bad. Her ultrasound evaluation suggested that her meniscus was pushed out of the joint and the ligaments that hold the meniscus in place were injured. However, her pain was near the scar. I decided to treat her with an initial prolotherapy treatment, but during the treatment, I tried to eliminate her pain before doing the actual injections. I was able to numb up the nerves around the knee and started to inject the scar. When that happened, her pain escalated. It was obvious to me that she didn't need a joint replacement immediately; she needed to have the nerves to her scar treated.

The medical history involves all the diseases that you have been diagnosed with, some of which may not be an issue anymore. Childhood asthma or bed-wetting may not have a profound effect on what we do, but it may open up other doors. For instance, late bedwetting, grinding of the teeth, and snoring during childhood are all abnormal. I was taught in medical school that gradually these things go away. Recently, I've learned that these are signs of sleep apnea, which you may still have. This is a health concern that might not seem important to reveal, but I like to address this as doing so will improve your health. This tangential process of getting more information during the interview is how I educate you in the many aspects of your health. You will thus need to bring a pen and paper.

Allergies are important. Some people are allergic to the anesthetic that I usually use. When this is an issue, I can use a different anesthetic. I use ropivacaine regularly because it is not toxic to platelets and stem cells.

Since the goal is to inject your own living cells into you, I don't want to injure them along the way. I avoid using Lidocaine or procaine, for this reason, because they are toxic to platelets *and* cartilage cells. They are typically combined with a steroid and injected into joints. As I treat you, if I know about it beforehand I will avoid anything that can cause you harm.

A seemingly-unrelated issue, such as gluten sensitivity, may change my recommendations for treatment. I avoid prolotherapy in these individuals, instead opting for treatment with platelet-rich plasma. The prolotherapy solution contains anesthetic, lidocaine, and dextrose sugar water. It is made from corn, manufactured or processed to make medical grade dextrose, in facilities that process other grains, such as wheat. I have noticed that in my patients with more severe gluten intolerance even a small amount of contamination will make their specific symptoms associated with gluten exposure worse.

I like to know all the medications and supplements you're taking. It's helpful to know why they were prescribed and by whom. The most common medications to avoid with any of the treatments that I offer are non-steroidal anti-inflammatory drugs (NSAIDS), such as ibuprofen, Aleve, and the like. Prednisone or steroids in any form, from eye drops to inhalers to pills, can also interfere with healing and should be avoided.

Other medications include the statins that are used to control cholesterol and some high blood pressure medications. Cipro, an antibiotic in a class called fluoroquinolones, has been associated with Achilles tendon injuries and should be avoided like all other antibiotics during treatment.

Family history is also part of the interview. It can be extensive and help guide decision-making. It's always concerning to me when someone has been diagnosed with fibromyalgia after another family member has been diagnosed, as if it is a hereditary condition. Perhaps it is, or perhaps the diagnosis was incorrect to start with. I have identified another reason for their pain more than once in my office. The issue may be that everyone is hypermobile, meaning that their joints have a larger arc of motion than normal. People with hypermobility, which can be inherited, have an issue with their collagen in their connective tissue. Sometimes the diagnosis can be Ehlers Danlos Syndrome (EDS), or it can be a spectrum with variations of increasing range of motion, affecting one or more joints. Usually in their childhood, these people can do the splits and are extremely flexible. They participated in gymnastics, dance, or ice-skating as children, which usually will worsen the condition. The treatment is any of the regenerative medicine procedures that I describe in the next chapter. The issue that is important here is that, although your family history is important, there is a chance that the diagnosis that you have may actually be treatable and you don't have to live with pain as a diagnosis of fibromyalgia suggests.

The social history usually involves whether you smoke, drink alcohol, or are married. For me, this is the time when I start to understand how committed you are to your health. This isn't a judgement time. There is no doubt that we all have our issues that we can improve upon. However, if your diet is not ideal, your ability to heal is not ideal. We know now that that you can alter the way your genes are turned on or off with dietary changes.

I fully understand how hard it is to prepare really healthy meals when you are in pain or busy. However, it is possible to make small changes along the way to get your body into the position of being more ideally suited to heal. The more vegetables there are in your diet, the more you can turn on your body's ability to reverse the effects of free radicals, which injure DNA. I have a scanner that uses state-of-the-art laser technology in the office to measure this. It's a wonderful tool to assist in understanding what your baseline ability to heal is.

The other aspect to the social history is what you love to do that gives you pleasure. I like to know your hobbies. I want to know if you can still pursue the gardening that you love. I also want to know what you do for exercise. If you are not able to exercise to the degree that you want or you alter that type of exercise so that you can still participate, that suggests that you have an injury that needs to be treated. Usually people who continue to exercise, avoiding things that hurt them, are the hardest people to convince that they need to be treated. To them, movement is life. I love that. I don't want to take that away, but long term, the injury only gets worse. It is possible to continue to exercise and to get treated at the same time. Many times, the exercises that you are avoiding will still need to be avoided in order to treat you. As you heal, and with some help from physical therapists or other exercise specialists, we'll get you back into the full body routine. The easiest people to treat are those that have just lost their ability to participate in the things they love. They recognize the injury, its effect on their sleep and emotional life, and they haven't lost hope. The people who are on disability with chronic pain or who have full-body pain have a harder time making decisions. Living with high levels of daily pain clouds your ability to think. Usually there are financial restrictions, too. I usually need help treating these individuals from a functional medicine doctor or naturopath.

In the next portion of the interview, we review lab work, radiographic reports, and the images.

Some people have had blood testing or saliva testing for their hormones. I am especially interested in these results, as I equate aging with a loss of hormones. Hormones assist with the body's ability to heal or recover from changes that normally happen to the DNA, affecting the cells. Another way of saying this is that we are always experiencing injury at the level of the DNA in the cell, but our body is invested in itself and has ways to repair these abnormal sequencings of DNA all the time. In childhood, this occurs rapidly, much faster than it does when we turn forty and the hormone levels have dropped. The hormones that I am interested in are the thyroid hormones (TSH, free T4, and free T3), DHEA-S, testosterone total and free, estradiol, progesterone, and vitamin D3. Labs usually establish normal levels by averaging out the results that the general population has at whatever age you are when you get the labs drawn. Effectively, as you age, they assume that normal is a lower number. There is research done to show that if you maintain hormonal levels in the high normal range, your ability to heal improves. The tissue in all parts of your body remains robust. The symptoms that are associated with loss of hormones may include fatigue, inability to maintain muscle mass, and depression/anxiety besides the expectant hot flashes, low libido, and weight gain. The lab's values should be checked, just like your cholesterol is tracked, at least once a year, more after starting the treatment with bioidentical hormones. I will discuss this further in Chapter 7.

Radiographic testing is a necessity. However, on x-ray, we know nothing about what occurs in the joint or the tissue around the joint. The MRI and ultrasound exams tell us more about these things. I perform an ultrasound exam of the joint, or area where you have pain, during your office visit, which offers an unique ability to evaluate the area. We refer to this as dynamic. Dynamic testing means that we can move a joint, stress a joint, or contract a muscle and see what happens as we look at the area with the ultrasound. X-ray or MRI, in contrast, are static ways to evaluate the area involved. X-rays provide a big picture view of the bones. We get obvious clues that there is an injury if the bone is fractured or broken and more subtle clues if there are spurs or boney growths. If the space between the joints is narrowed and there are spurs at the joint, we call this arthritis. This can be rated as mild, moderate, or severe. However, on x-ray, we know nothing about what occurs in the joint or the tissue around the joint. The MRI and ultrasound exams tell us more about these things.

The MRI is what we use to evaluate cartilage. In the knee, for example, there are two types of cartilages: articular cartilage, which is a layer that covers the bones at the ends where they meet the next bone, and the meniscus, which is a fibrocartilage. The MRI can evaluate both of these types of cartilage. Everyone above the age of thirty-five has meniscus cartilage tears or fraying. If you have knee pain and get an MRI, the most frequent recommendation that a surgeon will make is to "trim" the cartilage. We know this because it is the most common orthopedic procedure in the nation. However, if this is normal wear and tear, we don't know that this is the cause of pain. And there is a reason that the meniscus is there, so if it is removed, what will happen next?

The meniscus has a role in offering nutrition to the joint. Its shape helps to guide the joint through its motion. When it is cut, the physics of how your knee moves or bends is changed. I think of it as an instantaneous change in the velocity and angulation of the joint. It is subtle when it is a small portion of the meniscus, but when it is a larger portion, I can feel it and see it occur as a person walks. The general issue with removing a small portion of the meniscus is that one meniscus surgery begets another meniscus surgery which begets a joint surgery. The meniscus is also a cushion between two bones, the femur (thigh bone) and the tibia (lower leg bone). When the meniscus is damaged (along with some of the other ligaments that hold the knee together) the two bones, femur and tibia, can come in closer proximity to each other, and when they contact each other, the articular cartilage can be damaged, which can be seen on an MRI.

The degree of articular cartilage is one way we decide what type of treatment would be ideal for you. The MRI also visualizes the structures that surround the joint, the muscles, ligaments, and tendons. Because the MRI takes static images or cuts in three different planes, physicians have to recreate what the joint looks like in 3-D. I prefer to view the images in two planes at a time with you and my skeleton (who adds the third dimension), so I can show you where the injury is.

Other injuries that are important to evaluate in the knee by MRI are the anterior cruciate ligament (ACL) and the posterior cruciate ligament (PCL). Damage to these ligaments can be treated with regenerative orthopedic medicine, as well. Other structures that are evaluated by MRI can also be evaluated by ultrasound. The medial collateral ligament (MCL), the lateral collateral ligament (LCL), quadriceps tendon, patellar tendon, patellar ligaments, nerves, and blood vessels are easily evaluated by ultrasound, which can see injuries that are smaller than what the MRI can detect and can see them as they are in the body, versus having to recreate the three dimensions.

Ultrasound, MRI, and x-rays are all tools to help assist with understanding what is going on in an area of the body. They should not be used to make decisions independent of the physical exam. This was something that was reiterated over and over in my sports medicine training. This is important because where someone experiences discomfort or pain may not be where the abnormalities are on an x-ray or MRI. If the reason behind pain is not treated, what is the point? I gave the example of the knee because knee replacements have statistically been reported to have been unnecessary sixty percent of the time they are performed. I have had a few patients who have undergone the tremendous risk of doing a knee replacement, only to have their original pain not addressed and have more limitations with pain and function after the surgery. This is not to say that TKR, total knee replacements, aren't an opportunity for some patients to regain their functional lives. The point is that the physical exam and the radiographic studies need to correlate and that some of the treatment options that I present later may abate the need for surgery or may improve the outcome.

The physical exam is a portion of the initial evaluation where your body is evaluated. I am an osteopath through and through. I believe that the body has an innate ability to heal *and* that the body is interconnected and can't be evaluated based on one joint or organ system alone. In the situation of tailbone pain, what we may find on examination may be different from one person to the next. I always evaluate someone walking, standing, sitting, and laying down. I look for symmetry in three planes. When you stand up, for example, I look directly at you for symmetry between shoulder height, shoulder blade position, clavicular attachment to the sternum, rib symmetry, spine straightness (the opposite being a scoliosis), pelvic height, knee cap position, and foot position. I evaluate you as you walk, bend over, side bend, and rotate.

Tailbone discomfort can come from the tailbone itself, or it can occur at the sacrum or at the sacroiliac joint, where the pelvis attaches to the sacrum. This area is complicated. The sacroiliac joint is the attachment of the spine (the sacrum being the lowest or most inferior part of the spine) to the legs. The femur or thigh bone is attached to the pelvis, which is important for protecting the inner contents of your belly, bladder, sexual organs, and intestines, as well as a huge network of blood vessels and nerves. This joint can get injured in a fall or a car accident (usually on the right side, as this is the leg that slams on the brake; the force is transmitted up the leg to the hip or SI joint) or during HVLA (High Velocity Low Amplitude) manipulation techniques that both chiropractors and osteopaths use to force joints back in place. Running repeatedly on banked roads can injure it—and most roads are banked to assist with water drainage. The injury can occur over decades and not as a single event. The injury can be a secondary injury during childbirth. I have no doubt in my mind that pregnancy and delivery can be injurious to the body; I experienced this myself. The ligaments that relax or are loosened by the hormone relaxin during the third trimester of pregnancy don't always go back to where they are supposed to. The effect of this natural process on how the body is held together with the hormonal changes can be profound. It's amazing to me that rehab is not considered necessary after delivery.

When evaluating you in a supine position (lying flat on your back), I look for leg length discrepancy, pelvic motion, spine position, and muscular tension. I do this in general for any joint or injury below the waist that I am evaluating. It gives me a baseline for what your normal is before we start treatment.

I usually evaluate each joint in certain positions. As sports medicine physicians, we spend hours in our fellowship year perfecting and understanding what maneuvers should be used to test each joint. We are likely the most proficient at doing these exams of any of the specialists who do orthopedic regenerative medicine. The osteopathic training has given my fingers the tactile or sensory input to know what normal healthy tissue feels like compared to injured tissue. The combination allows for the ability to discern if injection therapy is needed on any one day.

Jane presented to my office after having PRP done to her elbows. She felt like she was progressing and had worn the prescribed braces to prevent re-injury after the treatment. She felt like she had injured the area again and was worried about the loss of muscle definition and strength that had occurred since her treatments four months prior. It was strange to me that she was experiencing so much discomfort. I did the exam and was able to provoke the pain. However, when I touched the tissue, it felt bound up. I used the ultrasound to evaluate the areas and very subtly, with movement of her wrist, I could see that the tissue at her elbow was bunching up. I felt the abnormal movement and proved it with ultrasound, knowing that the treatment that I gave her with PRP should have resulted in healing. I used my osteopathically trained hands and started to unwind and lengthen the fascia. This is when my right brain turned on. I followed the tissue, letting the resistance in the tissue guide the treatment. Over the course of an hour, we worked together, Jane guiding me with verbal cues of what she felt needed to be treated, and we got her out of discomfort and pain. I love it when a person's body is ready to receive and I become a conduit to healing.

The last part of the initial visit is when we review what was discussed in the interview, what was noted on laboratory and radiographic testing, and what was done in the physical exam to determine what treatment options can be done to get to your goal. As you know, I specialize in orthopedic regenerative medicine, using injections to treat nerves, muscles, fascia, tendons, and joints. However, as I've indicated before, osteopathic manipulation may also come into play. We make sure that we correlate what you are feeling symptomatically with what I feel on exam and see on radiographic images. I will make recommendations based on your goals.

For Paul, he could not have surgery, as his heart would not withstand the use of anesthesia. He understood the risk that thousands of people a year who die while getting their knees and hips replaced each year didn't. He was borderline diabetic and had already received his share of steroid shots in his knees, which caused his blood sugars to elevate for weeks but did not help him continue to walk. His goal was to stand and to walk around his house. He was in his seventies and had a wonderful, happy disposition. He had read about the benefits of platelet-rich plasma and wanted to pursue treatment. He was treated both inside the joint and to the many ligaments, capsule, and fascia attachments around the joint, as well as to the sensory nerves that supply the knee with nourishment through their interaction with the local blood supply and assist with healing in a way that was not taught to me in my formal training. Three PRP treatments later, he was walking.

Physical therapy was an essential component to getting his gluteal muscles firing better to help stabilize his large frame so that his quadricep muscle could assist with movement and not tighten in an effort to support his leg. Quadricep dominance is a term we use for people whose quadriceps are used incorrectly as a way to generate motion or hip stability. It happens in elite athletes and recreation athletes alike. It is a biomechanical issue, a postural issue, and a bad habit that I believe can lead to injury at the knee or any joint. Understanding an injury and what caused it is the premise behind being a sports medicine doctor.

Paul, in his youth, was a football player and used weight lifting throughout his adult life to keep his legs strong. This allowed him to be successful as an athlete but also created the habitual firing pattern that probably caused additional wear and tear of his knees. We needed this pattern to be retrained during physical therapy. Hypertrophy, or contraction of the muscle, is one aspect of getting strong. Another aspect is keeping the muscles and fascia pliable and lengthened. This is especially important as we age. Yoga is one way to do this; dynamic stretching is another.

At the end of the visit, I will suggest an individualized plan of treatment. There is no algorithm. It is a dynamic plan, meaning that options for treatment may change as we peel away the layers of the onion, the onion being your injury or the cause of your pain. I've heard many practitioners who do body work describe this phenomena where the original injury as you may know it is really a manifestation of other previous injuries. Eventually, we would like to get to why the injury occurred and treat that. Examples of why an injury occurred usually involve correcting postural habits, like the way you hold your head when you are reading the computer screen or the way that you stand or walk. Correcting muscle imbalances through physical therapy comes into play. Working with an athletic trainer or coach to correct movement patterns is important. Correcting foot position, especially during athletic pursuits, with arch support or orthotics or the right shoe is important. As we age, the position of our head as we try to accommodate for visual changes is important. I take what I hear you say, what I see you do, and what I feel on examination and the laboratory and radiographic tests to make decisions with you on where to start treatment and then adjust as needed as we go along. It's a process. In most cases, your injury took time to develop and will take time to heal. Since it is your body, I want you to feel welcomed to treat it. We are in this together.

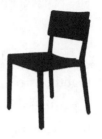

Chapter 6

REGENERATIVE ORTHOPEDIC MEDICINE TREATMENT OPTIONS

I t's decision time! What will be the best way to treat you? Your goal is my goal. In a previous chapter, my three-tier approach to orthopedic regenerative medicine was introduced. In this chapter, we'll discuss prolotherapy, platelet rich plasm, and stem cells in much more detail. I will discuss them as if they are distinct separate options, but in reality, we use a combination of these.

I'd like to introduce you to a few concepts first. These concepts are not widely understood by most doctors. What is taught in school from grade school through medical school is that the bones are the primary framework of the body. They are absolutely the framework, but they are not what holds the body together. To illustrate this to my patients, I show people my office skeleton. If it weren't for the screws connecting the bones, it would literally fall apart. Our bodies are held together by soft tissue or connective tissue, which includes muscles and their tendons, joint capsules, ligaments, and fascia.

Ligaments exert a compressive effect over a joint, meaning that when they are tight, the joint separates. This is hard to imagine and counterintuitive if you are thinking about a single attachment on one side of the joint. However, the joint is made up of a bone on both sides and has a joint capsule around it. There are ligaments, whose fibers weave into the joint capsule, along with tendon fibers, which attach muscle to bone. This creates a 360-degree covering around the joint. It's an ingenious basket-weave design. The fibers interweave with each other at various angles. When the fibers are nice and equally taut, there is a compressive effect across the joint that separates each bone from the other. Another way that you can think about this is with a Chinese finger toy. When you put a finger into either side of the toy, which is made in a basket-weave pattern, and pull, you will not be able to remove your fingers from the toy, but you can bend it like a young sapling. However, if you push your fingers together, the redundancy of the side walls of the toy between your fingers allows you to slide them across each other in a perpendicular fashion. It is this sliding that is abnormal that causes deterioration of the joint. I have a video on my Facebook page that illustrates this.

The concept that is important to understand is that joint arthritis is a consequence of abnormal movement in a plane of motion that is not supposed to happen. Injuries, that lead to arthritis, most commonly develop where ligament, tendon, joint capsule, and fascia attach to the bone. This is not to say that there aren't injuries that happen directly to the muscle. These do happen, but I look at the "welds" where muscle tendon attaches to bone or the tendon attaches to muscle as the more common location of the injury.

In the case of the tailbone, there is perhaps the largest and strongest network of ligaments in the body, connecting the pelvic bone to the sacrum (the tailbone being the most inferior, or lowest portion, of the sacrum). The tailbone can be dislodged or dislocated, which can be treated by someone trained in osteopathic medicine. Most likely, there is injury to this massive ligament structure that supports the SI joint. A common manifestation of this is an unequal leg length that can be corrected with adjustments. If these corrections don't hold, I will encourage you to stop the adjustments if they are done under any force and to pursue one of the three tiers of orthopedic regenerative medicine described below.

Now that you understand the concept behind what causes the injury, the treatment of any of these tiers of regenerative medicine occurs at the weld first. The long-term success of these regenerative medicine procedures occurs when the treatment is directed at the weld. There are regenerative medicine practitioners who will just treat the joint with a single injection. This is not enough.

In the next section, I will discuss the three major tiers of orthopedic regenerative medicine treatments. Each of these treatments encourages your body to heal. Prolotherapy is the entry level treatment. It requires more treatment sessions, however the recovery between treatments is relatively fast. Platelet-rich plasma is a stronger version of prolotherapy. It is used in moderate to severe injuries or for people who want to get better more quickly. Usually three to four treatment sessions are needed. Bone marrow stem cells are used in severe injuries after platelet-rich plasma has been used to start the healing process. Bone marrow stem cells encourage repair of damaged tissue. Usually only one treatment session is needed. The benefit is ongoing over the course of a year.

Prolotherapy

The first tier consists of the age-proven treatment called prolotherapy. It uses dextrose, sugar water. The concept behind prolotherapy that you need to understand is that the needle causes a small injury at the bone, from which the body has to heal. As I mentioned before, the injection occurs where a ligament, tendon, or fascia attaches to the bone. This small injury drives your body into healing mode.

When I am learning about you, I ask you to mark where you are experiencing pain on a body diagram, which helps me figure out what is causing your pain by the referral patterns that you have. For instance, the ligaments in the low back and sacrum have referral patterns in the leg, which may overlap with a sciatic nerve referral pattern with certain distinctions. Ligament referral patterns from the back will skip the knee, meaning that if you experience a referral of pain into your leg from a ligament, the pain is not perceived at the knee but rather above and below it on the leg.

If you come to me, you will likely experience prolotherapy, a cost-effective, precision-based treatment that I use initially on nearly everyone. The injury that is created with the needle, encourages platelets to migrate to the area. The platelet function is to clot the blood to stop any bleeding. The platelets lyse, or break open, releasing growth factors. This is a general term to describe what is generated next. Growth factors are honing molecules. They tell the body what to do in a systematic way. Some growth factors help to establish a blood supply to the injured tissue. Any tissue that has been injured for greater than six weeks does not have an adequate blood supply. This has been proven with biopsies of these areas in the past. Without a prolific blood supply to the area, the tissue (ligament, tendon, muscle, bone, or any other part of your body) will degrade or die. So the first step in healing an injury is to make more blood vessels. We call this neo- (meaning new) vascularization. This is an intrinsic occurrence when an injury occurs in the body that can be stopped or prevented with the use of anti-inflammatory medications. Growth factors also start to hone or encourage other things to come and repair the area, effectively building it back together. Amino acids, the smallest unit of protein, are these building blocks, which is why protein is a necessary part of the diet when you are healing.

Growth factors stimulate hormones and other growth factors in a series of reactions that are automated. There are many different types of growth factors, some you may have heard of, such as interleukins or cytokines. Some turn on and some turn off processes. This is happening in a microscopic world. I imagine it is like an ant hill or a bee hive where there is a lot of activity that looks chaotic as an outsider, but within the populations each ant or bee has a specific job that it is programed to do.

There is another concept that I want to reiterate. Prolotherapy invites all the wonderful growth factors to the injured area to encourage normal healing. Normal healing is organized. Scars that cause pain, on the other hand, are not composed of normal organized tissue. During this process, we are not scarring down tissue. Scar tissue is normally de-vascularized, meaning it doesn't have a good blood supply. That is why nerves as they try to repair themselves can't grow through this tissue. The tissue that is repaired has a blood supply, is supple, moves easily, and is not painful. The goal with prolotherapy is to change the micro-environment and promote healing.

Each needle injection, no matter what is being injected, is precisely placed with the help of an ultrasound machine, which allows for visualization of the body part and the needle. The imaging is done in real time, as if it were a movie not a snapshot. The needle is guided to its destination, and I watch whatever substance I inject through the entire process. The ultrasound is used during the entire treatment process to identify the injured areas. This is called ultrasound-guided injection therapy. I have become skilled at holding the ultrasound probe with one hand and injecting with the other, visualizing the process, which allows me to avoid blood vessels and nerves and other structures like lungs or other organs. It improves my precision and reduces the risk of other injury and also allows me to see what is happening as I inject so that I can make appropriate decisions along the way. An example of this occurred with the injection of what I thought was a simple tennis elbow. When I injected, what I injected did not stay where it was supposed to. It leaked out, exposing a tear that was compressed or deflated initially. With observance of the injection with ultrasound, the diagnosis changed from an injured tendon to a torn tendon, and I had to change the treatment. I added something to help clot the platelets so that they would stay in the tear and help glue it together. The use of ultrasound became crucial to doing the correct treatment. It is important to image while treating to ensure that the diagnosis and treatment rendered are correct so that you get better.

The reason why I usually start with prolotherapy as the initial regenerative orthopedic medicinal procedure is because there are other structures that induce pain that are treated at the same time. We typically will get muscle releases or twitches during the initial treatment. The muscle tightness develops as a consequence to the ligaments being injured. When ligaments aren't supporting the joint correctly or the tendon is injured, muscles whose job it is to move you through space, the mobilizer muscles, try to pick up the slack. Literally, they pick up the slack by tightening up. They shorten and go into spasm. I can see where these muscle twitches occur with ultrasound as I inject. If the twitch occurs within the muscle as my needle passes through it, I proceed with the prolotherapy. However, if the twitch occurs at a fascial layer, I think "nerve" and will treat the nerve to the area in addition to the prolotherapy.

Prolotherapy treats the cause of these myofascial pain syndromes ("myo" referring to muscle and "fascia" of course referring to the fascia, which envelopes muscles and the bundles that compose muscles). As the initial regenerative orthopedic medicine treatment, ultrasound-guided prolotherapy treatment allows for further diagnosis of the injury while treating it. It helps to create a more global understanding of where your pain is coming from. Additionally, it allows you to experience what these injection treatments feel like and better prepare for treatment with platelet-rich plasma and stem cell treatment if that is the goal. Many millions of people have healed from prolotherapy. It does take more treatments than the PRP that I will describe next, but I have seen the benefits in terms of pain reduction and improved function in many people, in comparison to before using the platelet-rich plasma or stem cells in my practice. As I provide prolotherapy treatment for you, there will be a drop in the number of twitches or trigger points. This is a sign of healing.

Platelet-rich plasma

The next treatment tier is platelet-rich plasma (PRP). It uses platelets from your own blood that are concentrated and placed in the same areas as would be treated with prolotherapy.

Anyone trained in prolotherapy will offer treatment with PRP in a similar manner, treating the injured area more comprehensively. Some people refer to this as PRP prolotherapy. The concept is that the full joint or injured area is treated in addition to the joint space.

The concept behind the use of platelet-rich plasma in regenerative orthopedics is the same as prolotherapy. With prolotherapy, the goal is to create an injury that the platelets that are in your body rush to. They stop the bleeding and send out honing devices or signals to encourage collagen growth and other growth factors to encourage blood vessel growth. PRP injections don't have to rely on platelets to rush to the area, as they are literally placed in the area at concentrated amounts, from which they orchestrate healing in the same way but this time with an army that is seven to nine times stronger than with prolotherapy. The limiting factor is the amount of platelet-rich plasma that you can make. With prolotherapy, I may inject up to 60 cc of prolotherapy solution to the lower back and pelvis to treat your tailbone pain. However, the total volume of PRP may be only 10 to 15 cc. I can take 60 to 240 cc of blood, centrifuge it, remove the red blood cells (RBCs) and most white blood cells (WBCs), leaving behind platelets and plasma. Plasma looks like highly-concentrated urine. It is a transparent yellow. Platelet-rich plasma is a combination of plasma and platelets. It is a translucent yellow. In general, most people's platelet level is about 130,000 to 330,000 per microliter (ml). After the RBCs are taken out, a second centrifuge is done, which separates the platelets from the plasma. We remove most of the plasma, thereby concentrating the platelets in a smaller volume—hence the name "platelet-rich plasma." We want to concentrate the platelets to seven to nine times your normal level for most of the injections that we do directly onto bone to get a platelet level of 1.5 million cells per milliliter (This is the most recent recommendation, which may change as more research is done). The final volume of PRP is dependent on how much blood we take from the start and what your platelet level is.

Because I may be limited by the final PRP volume, I plan ahead and inject the most injured areas with PRP first. If there are other areas to treat, I will use the platelet-poor plasma, the leftover plasma that does not have platelets but has tons of growth factors. I regularly treat other things like nerves, scars, and fascia that would benefit from the growth factors. Sometimes, I will treat with a combination of PRP to the most injured areas and prolotherapy to the other areas. Prolotherapy allows for the joint or injured area to be treated more comprehensively.

Bone Marrow Stem Cell

The third tier of regenerative medicine that I offer is bone marrow stem cells (BM). I reserve this treatment for more severely injured areas. However, not all injured areas are candidates for bone marrow stem cells. For example, someone who has an effusion, or fluid in the knee, may not be a candidate for BM if, after I drain the fluid, it keeps coming back. However, they may become a candidate if the fluid in the knee does not reaccumulate with PRP treatments. I want to ensure some healing of the cartilage before offering a more robust treatment. This occurs in a two-fold way. As you may remember, the PRP changes the stability of the joint when the ligaments, tendons, joint capsule, and fascia are treated and start to tighten. This changes the wear pattern in the joint, which is also injected with PRP. It is this two-fold treatment that affords you the best benefit to healing.

For most people who can't sit and have tailbone pain, the ligamentous structures are what are injured, and we might not need to treat with bone marrow stem cells at all.

The difference between bone marrow and PRP has to do with what is introduced into the area. PRP encourages the process of healing. During this process, stem cells may also migrate to the area and assist with the last stages of healing. I suspect that there are stem cells in the PRP preparation too, as stem cells circulate in the blood. The way that the treatment is done is similar, but the process of collecting bone marrow stem cells is different. Bone marrow stem cells are obtained from the pelvis. I use ultrasound in my office to visualize the bone. The portion of the bone from which the bone marrow is taken is marked. This is done sterilely, removing the chance for infection. Bone marrow, which looks like blood, is removed carefully from four or five spots on either side. The stem cells that exist in the bone marrow lie close to the outer wall of the bone, known as cortical bone. For this reason, a few donation spots are needed in order to obtain adequate amounts of bone marrow stem cells. This is different than in other medical specialties where bone marrow is donated for a bone marrow transplant. Usually in these situations, a large amount of bone marrow is taken from one spot. Prior to removal of the area, the area is anesthetized. During the procedure, you should not feel pain, rather a deep ache that feels like something is being sucked out, which it is. It lasts just a moment and is easily tolerated.

Bone marrow stem cells need to be processed in a sterile hood and through a centrifugation process to remove small boney chips, fat, and other substances. Bone marrow stem cells are used to inject into joints, into bone that is injured, and into tissue that needs more help with healing. As discussed before, pre-treatment with prolotherapy and/or PRP is done to get a joint ready for these powerful cells to do their job.

Fat is another area that can be used. There are stem cells in fat, but to isolate them requires quite a process or requires use of an enzyme called collagenase. Since the FDA does not recommend either the extensive multi-step processing or the use of collagenase, I have chosen not to isolate stem cells from fat. Rather, fat can be used as a filler or scaffolding. This is how it is used in cosmetics. Fat gives contour to the body. In orthopedic regenerative medicine, fat is used to fill in tears or holes or give structure to something that is injured. The risks occur with the removal of fat. This is usually done in the buttock, belly, or back, where there is more padding. Very thin people may not have a good donation site. In order to obtain the fat, I numb up the tissue really well. Epinephrine is mixed with anesthetic to reduce the chance of bleeding. Time is taken to allow everything to get numb. Then the fat is carefully removed with a long thin instrument with a lot of holes connected to a syringe, avoiding any injury to the abdominal wall or the organs beneath it. It is sucked into the syringe. Currently, I use an EmCyte centrifuge to process the fat, bone marrow, and PRP. The system is approved by the FDA and allows for a consistent way to get the desired amount of end product while eliminating much of the possibility for human error. It allows smaller offices with less staff to do more advanced treatments.

Although using these stem cells and growth factors has the potential to improve or possibly repair an injured joint or tissue, advertising that they can cure a disease or cure your arthritis, tailbone pain, or other injury is not allowed by the FDA. As of yet, we don't have proof that they can cure. Part of this has to do with the fact that each and every one of us is unique. Our injuries are unique, our genetics are unique, and our ability to heal is unique. What makes us unique may be our psychological or spiritual belief system, or our nutrition, or the degree of injury at the time that treatment is rendered. In any case, if we can't repeat the same treatment and get the same result most of the time, it's really hard to say that the treatment cures. This isn't to say that it doesn't work. There are studies to that are long term that have shown that people treatment with regenerative orthopedic medicine procedures are doing well after their treatments. The goal is to set the right expectation for you. We will take the time to do this together.

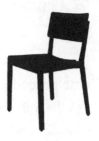

Chapter 7

WHAT CAN I DO TO IMPROVE THE SUCCESS OF BEING TREATED?

In the previous chapter, I described ways that I could treat you with prolotherapy, PRP, and stem cells to get you up and going again. This is what I can offer you, but it is not enough to achieve your goals. In this chapter, I will review other ways to improve your outcome. Some of the recommendations, such as dietary changes, may not be easy. I don't expect that you will make all the changes at once. It's too hard to do that for yourself, let alone to also attend to the individual needs of your family. I get it. Sometimes we start with supplements and gradually add the dietary changes as your energy improves. I will go over a few major areas that improve your success with the regenerative medicine procedures.

We recognize that people, as they age, develop diseases and injuries that don't heal. We think that is normal. However, there are cultures or sectors of the world where there are people who live longer. The author Dan Buettner, who wrote *Blue Zones,* spoke about the things that he identified in these populations that he studied. Interestingly, a vegetarian diet or a diet low in meat was one of the factors. Another aspect that was important was that these populations walked every day to do their daily errands. They lived where they could walk to the grocery stores. I love this concept, which correlates with the goal of 10,000 steps a day that other organizations have encouraged. A few other identifiers in these communities with people who lived past one hundred years old was that there was a religious or spiritual belief and a sense of service to other people. I love all these concepts. If I were to put it into other words, nutrition, daily exercise or activity, a loving supportive community, and a sense of purpose for the greater good have been shown to improve your lifespan.

Personally, the quality of that lifespan is really important to me. In the situation of injury or pain, it can be a struggle to try to encapsulate these things while juggling work, other stressors, and the kids and family life. The goal is to get you up and going again, and although I may not be able to counsel you through this, we've got to bring the appreciation or gratitude and joy back into our lives. Sometimes the struggle that is occurring is an opportunity to grow, and I can help you with the physical aspect of improving function and pain, but the spiritual aspect of how you see yourself is the process that you will journey through along the way. I'll be there, no doubt. I can feel the energy that you emit and may address these issues as we get to know each other.

There are so many recommendations about nutrition out there. It's hard to figure out what works for you. My expertise is not nutrition, but nutrition is one of my favorite topics to talk about, and I love to eat. General concepts that I think are relevant are that you are what you eat, meaning what you choose to fuel your body with affects the body's ability to heal. Anything processed has additives and preservatives or has been irradiated or altered to give it a shelf life. As I mentioned before, these are chemicals that can cause changes to your DNA. The more your body is exposed to them, the more it has to work to fix the changes that occur. Without the right nutrients, which include vitamins and minerals, the body is unable to do this. Organic fresh fruits and vegetables of all colors, in general, are a good general concept of healthy choices to eat. There should be a portion with every meal. Of course, there are outliers to every situation, such as food allergies, but this should apply to eighty to ninety percent of the population. I like to eat what is in season, as the microorganisms that live in the soil provide a benefit for intestinal health. The recommendations are seven to nine fruit and vegetable servings a day in their original form (raw) or cooked at a temperature less than 400 degrees. If you feel that you need to cook them in a fat, make sure the fat is stable at higher temperatures.

Spices and herbs have an innate way of not only providing flavor but also being medicinal. Make sure that they are not irradiated and throw them away if they lose their color or expire. If you look at ancient cultures and cook using the same variety of spices or herbs, there is a wisdom associated with this.

Organic, non-GMO (genetically modified organism) grains in smaller quantities are likely beneficial if your intestinal health is good. If you have what is now termed as leaky gut though, this increases the size of particles that are absorbed into the lymphatic and blood systems, which can be irritants and cause any number of symptoms. Many people can experience pain as a consequence of consuming gluten or other substances in grains. In situations where you are not absorbing nutrients correctly, what you eat may need to be adjusted or eliminated. This is a situation where working with a doctor, such as a naturopath or functional medicine doctor, may be important. I have found that an Ayuredic cleanse for two weeks twice a year has improved and repaired my digested system.

Seeds and nuts are a great source of healthy fat.

Organic meat, sustainably farmed without antibiotics and exposure to other chemicals, are a necessary part of some people's diets. Typically, in the American culture, especially with men (no judgment here), the diet leans heavily toward meat. While getting treated with anything that requires you to heal, it is important to have good sources of protein. This can be done with a vegetarian diet that has lots of beans, too. The amino acids necessary to build the body back together are found in protein. Meat is the easiest way to obtain this. However, most Americans get more than an adequate amount of protein in their diets.

What is not obtained in your diet can be obtained in supplements. It is important to get the supplements from a medical- or pharmaceutical-grade supplier because it is possible to buy supplements that have nothing in them that is beneficial. Supplements are not an industry that is regulated, although the state of California does have more stringent regulations for fish oil and perhaps other supplements than national standards. Our bodies often need mineral supplementation to offset the poor quality of most of the soil in this country. I provide general recommendations about what minerals are needed and typically encourage the use of a multimineral and vitamin combination.

Vitamins are necessary, especially if your diet is lacking in the seven to nine servings of fruit and vegetables. I suggest use of higher doses of vitamin C (1000 mg/day or more) as it has been found to have a profound effect at the cellular level, in terms of repairing cellular damage. Glucosamine, chondroitin, and MSM supplements have also been shown to provide protection of the joints. Vitamin D3 is actually a hormone that can be checked in the blood. Levels between sixty to eighty iu/day have been shown to be ideal for healing. If you are below these levels, the recommended dosing can be between 2000 iu to 5000 iu a day of vitamin D3. Fish oil at doses above 2500 mg to 3000 mg a day is also beneficial in a number of ways. I suggest that, whatever supplement that you choose to use, you find out what their rancidity level is (this determines how fresh it is) and what their PCB level is. PCBs are the smallest plastic particles that litter the sea. Fish consume them. I believe the California standard is less than 9 ppb, and there are companies that have less. The benefit of taking a fish oil supplement is offset if the concentration of PCBs are high. Fish oil may increase post-treatment bruising, as it is a blood thinner at higher doses. I recommend that most people take fish oil; however, I have been encouraging people to not use it three days before and the day of treatment.

Medications can have adverse effects in healing. Non-steroidal anti-inflammatory drugs (NSAIDs) interrupt healing and destroy the intestinal lining. They are responsible for many people dying each year due to complications from their use. These medications include both over-the-counter (OTC) and prescription medications. Advil, Aleve, Celebrex, naproxen, and Mobic are all examples of these medications. These need to be stopped at least two weeks before any of the regenerative procedures and should not be used after, during healing. Prednisone and other prescription steroids, in the forms of injections, eye drops, pills, inhalers, suppositories, or creams also should be stopped during the same time period. Aspirin at low dose if prescribed by a physician for a specific ailment may be continued. Bruising will occur though.

The concept behind the reason why these medications need to be stopped is your body heals normally through an inflammatory process. This process occurs in a temporal manner, meaning that it is orchestrated by time. Each sequence of events that is required in order to get normal healing occurs in a time-driven manner. The body knows what it needs to do to get the job done. When the healing that is supposed to occur on day three is interrupted by use of one of these medications, for the length of time that the medication is functioning in your body, no healing occurs. Then the body picks up at the time that it was supposed to and a layer of healing that occurs on day four follows the foundation laid down on day two. What was supposed to occur on day three is missing. This is a simplified version of what happens, but you get the idea that healing occurs in layers. It is a process that takes time. When the healing is incomplete because one of these medications is used, the tissue is not as strong and more likely to get injured in the future.

Other medications that also impair healing are the cholesterol-lowering medications and ACE-inhibitor class of medications for blood pressure. Cholesterol-lowering medications in the HMG-CoA class include Lipitor (atorvastatin), Zocor (simvastatin), and other medications whose generic name ends in "-statin." I encourage the use of the CoQ10 supplement. CoQ10 functions like a mineral. Its presence is required in order for the liver to process the medications. Other medications that need to be addressed include blood thinner medications, such as Coumadin, which should be held for three days prior to treatment because of the increased chance of bleeding with injection treatments. I recommend working with the doctor that prescribed these medications to adjust or hold the medications while treatment and healing is occurring. I will help to facilitate this conversation with your doctor.

Osteoarthritis of the knee is very common. This is different than the normal age-related wear and tear that we all have. This is not to say that surgery is bad. The point is that we need to consider and use research to guide our treatment. This is also the case with use of steroid injections into any joint. There is plenty of research on patients, similar to you, that shows that steroid injections are detrimental to joints. They accelerate cartilage breakdown, leading to osteoarthritis. The definition of osteoarthritis involves the breakdown or injury of the cartilage and bone. Why would you want to pursue treatment that guarantees further injury to the joint that you are trying to protect? This is the present medical model. This is what your insurance company will pay for.

Many times, by the time I see patients they have already received a steroid shot into the joint. It is the standard treatment taught in medical schools and used in major university hospitals and orthopedic clinics. It may have been the only thing that was offered to you besides surgery. This is a situation where what has been researched and studied lags behind what is incorporated into everyday practice of medicine. When steroids are used anywhere in the body, they may help with pain and swelling in the short term, but since they interfere with healing, they usually don't help in the long term. Corticosteroids come in a few forms; some can crystalize and also cause injury to the cartilage. In general, steroids weaken and thin tissue. An injection can do this at the area, leaving a white coloration to the skin and a dimple if the concentration of the steroid is high and some of it leaks from the needle to the tissue under the skin as the needle is taken out of the area.

Steroids affect blood sugar. When I worked as a family doctor, I would send my patients with diabetes to be evaluated for their knee or back pain. They would get a steroid shot, and I would manage their high blood sugars for the next month, having to add additional medications. These patients always told me that they were told that the local steroid injection would not affect their blood sugar. Perhaps that is what was taught to these doctors, but that is definitely not what I saw.

The other big effect that steroids have on the body is their effect on the body's own ability to make native corticosteroids. This affects how you feel and function. Because corticosteroids are hormones, the effect may be variable. In some cases, you feel fatigued. In other cases, it may be that your bones get weaker. You may be more susceptible to fractures in the spine, called compression fractures. This is not an uncommon finding with people who are on prednisone, a corticosteroid in a pill form, for extended periods of time. This is painful. The use of bioidentical hormones to reverse the aging effect of loss of hormones can be useful to treat compression fractures and thinning bones. This is not to say that I don't use them. Physiologically, very small doses of steroids can be helpful. Regenerative orthopedic medicine offers ways to provide treatment without causing more disease. It may be uncomfortable to receive and heal from these treatments, but it is an extremely safe and comprehensive approach to halting arthritis development and possibly reversing disease without side effects from medications or surgery, including anesthesia risks, scar development, allergies to metals in the joint replacement, and any of the other risks that are on the consent form that you sign immediately before you get surgery. Sometimes the use of the regenerative orthopedic medicine options can be used prior to surgery to improve your outcome. Usually, though, I see patients after surgery, when they still experience pain or have function loss.

Hormones, such as thyroid, Vitamin D3, DHEA-S, testosterone, progesterone, and estrogen, start to decline with age. I like to talk about optimizing these during our appointment. Bioidentical hormones definitely help with the recovery and healing process. You may respectfully decline them or choose to obtain them from another provider. I'm good with whatever decisions you make as long as you know that healing is faster with them. There are other benefits to these hormones, such as an improved sense of wellbeing, improved sleep, better energy, prevention of cognitive decline, heart disease, and stroke with age. The issue with deciding whether or not to treat with bioidentical hormones is a shift in what you know and understand about them. If you assume that diseases that occur with aging are normal and likely will happen to you, then bioidentical hormones are not for you. However, there is a lot of research evidence that suggests that they are safe if you consider a few things. The most important consideration is that the hormones that you take have the same exact chemical structure as those that exist in nature. This is what is meant by bioidentical. Progesterone is not the same as its chemically altered counterpart, progestin. Estradiol is not the same as conjugated equine estrogen from horse urine. There are nuances and different ways that different doctors prescribe them. It is harder to tailor doses in women, as there are more female hormones to adjust. Men are easy. They want testosterone. They know they feel great on it. It needs to be monitored, but the decision to be treated is easier for them.

In general, Provera and Premarin, pills that are prescribed for hormone replacement in women, both should be avoided. I suspect that many of the birth control pills that are progestins versus progesterone based should also be avoided. They have been developed and patented by the pharmaceutical companies because the chemical structure has been altered. It is this change in chemical structure that our bodies do not know how to process, similar to what is happening with GMO food. The human genome cannot figure out ways to deal with the changes that chemicals have on our bodies when it is consistently exposed to chemicals or irritants all the time, meaning that if there was only one chemical that altered our genetics or our DNA, our body might be able to repair the gene that was affected easily, but in this day and age, our bodies are being exposed to food irritants, medication irritants, environmental irritants, EMS irritants (waves generated by Wi-Fi and cellular transmission of signals), sunscreens, and beauty products that have chemicals and can be irritants. The point of this is not to scare or overwhelm you, but rather to empower you to learn more about the benefits of hormones and consider bioidentical hormones if you choose to pursue them with me or another provider.

For me, the key to understanding treatment with bioidentical hormones is really learning how to read medical research. Sometimes what doctors understand from hearing about research is very different than what was printed in the research paper. It's similar to the telephone game that we played as children. The original message becomes totally convoluted as the message passes from one person to the next.

Hormones also monitor our sympathetic and parasympathetic nervous system. The sympathetic nervous system governs our fight or flight response to stress or dangerous situations. Many people live in this state of being on guard all the time. The parasympathetic system, on the other, hand is calming. I recognize the value of breathing, meditation, yoga, craniosacral, and acupuncture treatments, which all encourage our parasympathetic system to turn on. I make an effort to participate in activities that are reflective and slow me down. The goal is to be present and enjoy the journey.

After the injections, you may feel a little weak or unstable. Perhaps this instability is the norm for you and why you came in. In both situations, a brace can help protect the joint while it is recovering and help place the joint in proper alignment to get it to heal correctly. There are ways that we can physically protect the joint from getting injured. I like to use well-constructed orthotics for ankle and foot issues and possibly for knee and hip issues if the ankle/foot position instability is leading to these other issues. This may involve using a brace for the knee, back, SI joint, elbow, wrist or thumbs. For example, your tailbone pain may be related to Sacroiliac (SI) joint dysfunction. An SI belt can be used to keep the SI joint from moving as much, retaining you in a more ideal position. Remember all these regenerative procedures cause a controlled injury from which you need to heal. Immediately following treatment, the area treated is weakened and more prone to injury. I want to protect the joint during this time period. In situations where we need regrowth of the cartilage, such as in the knee, we may use a brace to correctly align the joint and to prevent further injury during the healing process. The shoulder is difficult to brace well; however, a sling works well to relieve the muscles from being used after treatment. The neck typically is not braced, as the neck muscles are so important to holding up the head and they quickly weaken when they are not used (for example, when a cervical collar is used; however, for a shorter time, less than 24 hours, a cervical collar may be needed to travel home to help stabilize and prevent injury). Braces can be covered by your health insurance, but usually there is a deductible that must be met. A deductible is an amount that your insurance requires you to pay before they start to pay. I can help assist you in getting high quality braces, although in some cases, an off the shelf brand can work fine. Usually crutches and slings are needed for only 24 hours but can be beneficial for an additional one to three days depending on the procedure that was done. Crutches can off-load or prevent pressure on a joint in the lower portion of the body to help protect the joint immediately after treatment. I think of it like ketchup on a hamburger. If the joint is loaded immediately after a treatment, everything within the joint is squished out, which may be exactly what we are trying to prevent, especially if the meniscus was treated in the knee.

Exercise is appropriate if it does not cause pain or discomfort during, immediately after, or the next day. In some cases, such as after knee replacement surgery, there will be pain related to the surgery, and it is necessary to participate in observed exercise to prevent the scar from limiting the range of motion (ROM) and to encourage tissue regrowth and correct muscle contraction patterns. For procedures in my office, you may experience some swelling and discomfort after the treatment, but the pain is much less comparatively to surgery. I will encourage you to move to keep the blood flow to the area. For shoulder injuries, avoiding exercise that will injure the shoulder is obvious. Swimming, for example, is not a great idea for exercise if your shoulder, elbow, or wrists are injured. Using a kickboard or participating in an exercise program in the water may be okay. On the other hand, with hip, knee, low back, foot, and ankle injuries, a water-based program and swimming with a pull buoy may be fine, while the treadmill would be counterproductive. Elliptical and cycling are both non-weight-bearing exercises and can be done for aerobic exercise while healing. I love it when you can get your heartrate up daily while healing. Scary movies and video gaming do not count!

Stabilization exercises are more important than strength-based exercises. With the proper physical therapy for recovery after these treatments, stabilization exercises are fundamental. Stabilization exercises can be static, meaning you hold a position, for example a plank. They can be more dynamic: a plank exercise on a ball or other uneven surface or one-armed or one-legged or while using elastic bands. Stabilization exercises can be abdominal core exercises, however there are core or stabilization exercises for every joint in your body. Usually there is a stabilizer injury that needs to be rehabbed at the center of the "onion."

When I worked at the University of New Hampshire in the Student Health Center, I had the opportunity to see a few of the football players with back pain. These are big Division I athletes. There were no x-ray findings, no disc issues, but they had pain. The old "no pain, no gain" saying may be the attitude of the coach or the trainers, but I've long since retired that thought. Pain is a sign that there is something going on. Since I couldn't recreate the pain with my fingers or by moving the athletes into certain positions, I asked one athlete to do a plank and raise one arm in the air. He could not. We addressed a few of his stabilizer muscles (psoas, multifidi, TVA) with exercises, which he did. When he came back, he quickly got into the plank position and showed me his progress. We started to add more exercises that he did on his own to maintain his body for the rigors of high-intensity university athletics. I wondered at what point this loss of core stability occurred. A few years after I took care of this football player, I figured it out. When my son went to kindergarten, he started to sit at a desk for most of the day. Prior to this, I could lift him over my head and hold him by his pelvis while he kept a straight airplane position. By the end of his first full year in school, he had lost this ability. Sitting is the culprit. As my son approaches his teenage years, I recognize that he needs to simultaneously develop both the stabilizing core system and the muscle hypertrophy needed for strength to prevent injury. Participating in athletics can do some of this; however, maintaining good posture throughout the day is also really important. With cues, he can do this, but if distracted, his posture slumps. I bring this up because poor posture starts young with prolonged sitting. It can be the start of an injury pattern, a habit that needs to be retrained.

Obviously, smoking is not great for healing. As mentioned before, neither is alcohol. Alcohol use has been shown to reduce circulating stem cell levels (in your blood), so it is not recommended after treatment.

Both can be part of a complex addiction cycle. Nicotine in whatever form causes your blood vessels to constrict or narrow, reducing the blood supply to areas that need oxygen to heal. Only three cigarettes total a day are needed to maintain the addiction. This can be done with a single inhalation and waiting ten minutes for the effect to get into the blood stream. The number of puffs that you take each day directly corresponds to increased risk of COPD or emphysema. You can decrease your risk by reducing your number of inhalations. Each inhalation, or drag, that you take in creates a microinjury to the little cluster of grapes called alveoli in your lungs where oxygen is absorbed into the blood stream. Over time, this cluster of grapes loses its elasticity, and the walls between the grapes break down, leaving not a cluster of little grapes but a sack. This sack has less surface area, to allow for absorption of oxygen. If you can prevent injury to these alveoli by reducing or eliminating the number of drags or inhalations that you take a day, you will reduce the development of emphysema, chronic bronchitis, pneumonias, and the need for supplemental oxygen as you age. Some find hypnosis can help you kick your habit. Acupuncture has been beneficial for others. Changing your habit to another one (not eating!) like exercise or developing a hobby that uses your hands or chewing gum with xylitol (to prevent sugar cravings and tooth decay) can be beneficial. You are not stopping smoking for me. You are doing it for you and the people who want to see you not suffer as you age.

Sleep is totally underrated. As we push ourselves to get work done, burning the candle on both ends, we compromise our sleep. Most people need eight hours of uninterrupted sleep. You are supposed to wake up refreshed, alert, and ready to go. I don't know about you, but I rarely have mornings like that. However, it is during sleep that we heal. If you can't sleep, it's a good idea to develop good sleep hygiene. With your children, turn off the electronics at eight p.m., avoid late eating, get into bed at ten p.m., avoid heavy exercise before bedtime, use your bed only for bedroom-related activities, and avoid watching TV, working, and reading in bed.

For many Americans, their other medical conditions can prevent them from healing. Diseases such as diabetes, heart disease, dementia, and cancers all fall into a group of disorders that occur as a consequence of chronic inflammation. This is different than the bit of inflammation that I cause with an injection that your body has to heal from. This is inflammation throughout the body caused by chronic irritation, likely that starts in the intestinal tract. All of these diseases are potentially reversible, depending on the time that you address them. This is not an area of expertise for me but these are situations that I recognize could compromise your ability to heal. Functional medicine doctors, naturopaths, or Ayurvedic providers can provide a great service to you by evaluating, treating, and monitoring these conditions differently than how I was taught in my training. There is so much more to treating disease than medications and surgery.

Because it matters to me that you get the best possible outcome, there are times where I won't treat or will delay treatment until you are evaluated by someone who can change the course of your disease proactively. If you are committed to your own health, I will be invested in your treatment. The last thing that I want to happen is to have you pay for a procedure that is not covered by your health insurance and that won't work for you if there are other things that need to be done first. I'm sure there are clinics that are happy to take your money and offer treatment in non-ideal situations, but this is not one of my goals.

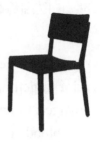

Chapter 8

WHAT CAN I EXPECT DURING TREATMENT?

You've committed to making a change in your pain! In this chapter, I will discuss what you need to do on the day of treatment to prepare for prolotherapy, PRP, or bone marrow stem cells.

First, I ask that you obtain the braces or orthotics that you need prior to treatment. Depending on where I inject, we want to prepare for healing by having the joint be in an ideal position for healing. I discussed the use of braces last chapter. The purpose here is to simply to remind you of the importance of having a brace or orthotic. Sometimes orthotics needs to be constructed, and you will have to wait for it. That is fine. Your treatment does not have to be delayed.

I have reviewed avoiding certain medications prior to getting treated. Some medications need to be changed to another medication that can do the same job (blood pressure), some medications need to be held (fish oil, blood thinners), and some medications need to be avoided for a minimum of two weeks before and six weeks after treatment (anti-inflammatory medications, steroids). It is important that there is an adequate amount of time prior to being treated to do these things in conjunction with your primary care provider.

In your situation, the tailbone injury, especially if it occurred during a car accident, has many areas that are injured, necessitating additional injections. There are many ligaments in the sacral area. There are muscles that attach to bones via tendons. Both the muscles and tendons can be injured. Nerves can be injured or entrapped. These all need to be treated. Remember the layer of tissue that envelops muscles, blood vessels, and nerves called fascia? This is the thin layer that surrounds a chicken breast that is difficult to cut through. It is distinctive from the muscle, which is easy to cut through. It is this fascia that allows muscles to slide across each other when they contract. It is also the fascia that can get adhered or stuck together and the cause restriction in movement that Rolfers treat with their hands. Massage therapists can also feel these restrictions, and physical therapists, osteopaths, and chiropractors have been trained to feel for them. I can see where the restrictions occur under ultrasound. These need to be treated. Scars need to be treated. These soft tissue structures all support joints. When injured, the SI joint moves too much and leg length can change. Adjustments help, but if they don't hold, it suggests that there is an injury to the other structures that hold the joint in place. They need to be treated in addition to the SI joint. We've discussed this before, but I am reiterating this purely to discuss expectations of the number of injections that occur during a pro-lotherapy injection session. There are many. It is not a single injection event. There can easily be thirty injec-tions, including the anesthetic to any injected area. This doubles when treating the back and pelvis.

One of the biggest concerns when treating anyone with any procedure that introduces something from outside the body to inside the body, such as a needle or a surgical device, is the risk of infection. We use gloves, sometimes masks, gowns, drapes, or covers over the area that we treat. This depends on how inva-sive or how intrusive the procedure is. If I inject into a joint, I want to take every precaution to avoid intro-ducing bacteria from your skin into your joint. When a joint gets infected, these bacteria are the ones that might grow. That is why a doctor washes and cleans the skin over the joint. This is why I use gloves, a cover

over the ultrasound probe, and sterile ultrasound gel. I will wash the skin after I use anesthesia and right before I inject. It's a process. These are things that instructors reiterated in medical school and residency, as I watched surgeries and later assisted with surgeries. I remember having to re-scrub after getting gowned up prior to surgery when my glove accidently touched something that was not sterile.

This is also important when the platelets, stem cells, and fat are processed. This is done in a hood, something that filters and circulates the air within it but is contained so that only the lab technician's hands are within it. Imagine a food bar at Whole Foods, where a glass panel separates your face from the food, lessening the chance that you can cough, sneeze, or breathe on the food. The hood is like that, with side walls and a small opening in front.

The treatment you receive should be done with you in a comfortable position, usually lying down. The equipment and positioning should be set up before the procedure. We use caution to eliminate, to the best of our ability, any infection by using clean or sterile techniques. The degree of sterility depends on the invasiveness of the procedure; bone marrow stem cell acquisition and fat need more sterility. A single joint injection needs less. An injection into the spinal column, such as an epidural, needs more caution taken.

If your body position needs to change and I help you, I will have to change my gloves and re-wash the skin over the area that I am treating. Most of this happens without you realizing what is going on. On occasion, there are people who talk with their hands and have to show me where they are experiencing discomfort by physically touching it. Although I try to prevent this from happening, it does occur, and we have to wash the area again. I'll let you know if this happens. I want you to be aware that these things that I do to avoid infection occur and are important in terms of improving outcomes.

Another area of interest for you is what we do while we are processing. There are ways to make PRP and isolate stem cells from the blood and bone marrow from scratch and from kits. The use of kits has made processing faster and reduces the risk of contamination but may limit what can be done because the volume used is preset. The FDA encourages the use of kits to reduce the risk of infection. This is especially the case when there is no hood to process the PRP in. The blood is not exposed to air at any time. The kits vary in expense, along with the cost of the particular centrifuge that is used. This has driven up the cost of the procedures, unfortunately. I am able to make PRP from scratch, too. I obviously do this in a hood. This increases the amount of PRP that I can make at a single time so that I can concentrate it more or so that I have more volume to inject. I need more volume when I treat the back, for example, or if someone wants more than one joint injected. The larger volume takes longer to process and requires someone who is trained more.

Another aspect that comes into play is what your platelet levels are prior to treatment. If your platelet levels are lower, then when obtaining the seven to nine times the concentration of platelets, we may have less volume to start with. It's helpful for me to keep track of all this information for research purposes, too. I find that the more I individualize the processing to achieve the desired concentration of platelets, the more consistent the outcomes are.

It's tough when someone doesn't get better as quickly or to the same degree as someone with the same amount of damage to a joint. We haven't perfected the outcomes of each of these procedures so that one hundred percent of the people we treat get one hundred percent better. Like all aspects of medicine, it is an art. Opportunities to further improve the orthopedic regenerative medicine specialty will be presented with each passing year. The specialty is growing; new advances are being made regularly. My goal is to continually improve what I am capable of doing in my office and become proficient in each skill that I develop while maintaining safety and adapting the treatment for each unique patient that I see. I love developing relationships with patients as we journey through the process together. Trying to solve or treat the cause of your physical pain or discomfort drives me.

So back to the procedure itself. After cleaning the area first with a combination of soap and alcohol, the ultrasound is used to identify the areas that will be treated, which are marked with a pen or use of an anesthetic injection. Anesthesia of the skin and deeper areas occurs next. Each time this occurs, you will experience the sensation of a needle prick through the skin. For some people, this is not an issue; for others, an anti-anxiety medication can be used twenty minutes prior to the procedure. For people who are needle-phobic or have more pain to start with, we can use nitrous oxide (laughing gas). If you need anti-anxiety medication or nitrous oxide, we can provide this for any of the procedures described here; just let me know in advance. It is important to me to allow time for the anesthetic to work and make sure you are numb before starting.

After the area is numb, the treatment starts. The first treatment is always the most difficult to gauge. You don't know what to expect during the treatment or after. If you are apprehensive during the treatment, sometimes you forget to breathe, which is the single most important thing that you can do to help yourself through the procedure. The injection onto bone feels like a buzzing sensation. It's uncomfortable but momentary. The goal with injecting is to just touch the bone with the needle; there is no stabbing of the bone. This is what makes it so elegant and precise. The part of the treatment that is most uncomfortable occurs when the muscle twitches when a trigger point is released. It catches you off guard. Removing these twitches that occur most predominately when the back and pelvis are treated with prolotherapy allows for an easier treatment session with PRP. It takes about thirty minutes to an hour to treat most joints. The use of ultrasound increases the time but also improves accuracy.

Throughout out the procedure or treatment session, I will ask how you are doing. Sometimes, I will ask you what you are feeling. Some people prefer to disassociate from their body with hypnosis, while others distract themselves with music that they play on their phones, while others are tuned in with what is going on. Sometimes I talk to help distract people. Some people want a play-by-play of what is happening, and I'll let them know. If you need a breather or a position change, let me know. This is not a rush. Some joints require that we change your position so that we can access the joint from multiple angles. The hip joint, for example, is treated while you're on your belly, on your side, and then on your back. We use bolsters or pillows to support your body in these different positions. We want you to be as comfortable and warm as you need to be during the treatment.

As I've mentioned, I usually offer prolotherapy as the initial treatment for most people. The benefit from my perspective is I can make a large volume of prolotherapy solution that I can use to treat many structures, including nerves, fascia, joint, ligaments, muscles, and tendons by altering the dextrose concentration. Sometimes an injury such as a tear does not reveal itself until the tissue is injected. When I notice the tear, I can prepare for the next treatment, altering what I inject and when. I will discuss this with you if it comes up. From your perspective, we can start to change your pain quickly. Trigger point releases can dramatically lower your pain within twenty-four hours. A nerve block can reduce your pain within the hour. I can use what you experience to determine what to do in the following treatment.

The biggest difference between prolotherapy and injections with PRP or stem cells is what to do to prepare prior to your arrival. Fat is a substance that appears in your blood after you eat a fatty meal. I don't want to inject this fat into you. For this reason, I recommend that you avoid fat for twelve hours prior to the treatment session. When I first learned to make or process platelet-rich plasma from the blood, I did two treatment sessions where we donated our blood. The second treatment session happened after lunch. Our lunch, which included only a little bit of fat in the mayonnaise of a chicken salad sandwich, clouded up some of the blood that was processed immediately following, making it difficult to separate it from platelets. It was interesting to me to see the vast difference in the amount of fat that appeared in the blood from one doctor to the next. I cannot predict for whom this will occur, so the general recommendation for everyone is to avoid fat. The other recommendation is to fast for four hours before blood, bone marrow stem cells, or fat grafts are taken.

Once you arrive at my office, we will immediately take your blood or extract your stem cells. There is a processing time that can take one to three hours. You may eat immediately after. Some people choose to bring their own food; others will walk into town to get food.

Platelet-rich plasma differs from prolotherapy because we are extracting your own blood, and there are fewer injections with PRP and/or stem cell treatments. The reason why there are fewer injections with PRP than prolotherapy is because we are limited by the amount of blood that you can donate. Typically, 60 cc to 240 cc (a cc is a milliliter) of blood is taken. About 500 cc are taken when you donate blood. This volume of blood is significant, which is why we want you to hydrate with about half your weight in ounces of water prior to the procedure. The goal is to concentrate your platelet number to seven to nine times what your normal number is. For someone who has a normal platelet count of 200,000/ml this works out roughly to be about 7 cc of PRP from 60 cc of blood. This limits the amount of available liquid (PRP) to inject. The treatment session usually lasts for an hour. I set up the treatment similarly to prolotherapy. I clean the area with alcohol and soap. A sterile cover is placed over the ultrasound probe. Anesthesia to the skin and deeper structures is used to numb up the area. The treatment is done similarly to prolotherapy; however, as mentioned above, fewer areas will be treated because of the limitation in volume. The injection with PRP onto bone burns and is uncomfortable. The area feels bruised. This can be momentary, or it can linger after the treatment for a bit. The area will look swollen and may bruise. Sometimes the amount of swelling prevents the use of a brace. Usually wrapping the joint with Coban or an ACE wrap helps.

Tier three procedures, bone marrow stem cells and fat to be used as a scaffold, are much more invasive procedures. This does not mean that they aren't safe; it means that I take more precautions to prevent infection. I acquire stem cells from bone marrow from the pelvic bone, as you are laying on your belly. I clean the area and sterilize, and then I use ultrasound to evaluate and identify the area from which all five of the samples on either side will be taken. The reason why five spots are used is to increase the yield of bone marrow-derived stem cells. I will mark each site with a pen. The skin is numbed, and then the bone is numbed, as is the area in between. You will experience the sucking sensation that I discussed previously when this is done. It's a weird sensation, lasting just moments. It should not be painful. I use a drill to assist me in obtaining the samples, as it is quicker for you and less cumbersome for me. We extract the bone marrow in a specific timing and amount from each area. The stem cells are located right against the hard, rigid outer bone called the cortical bone.

After the samples are taken, I place a compressive dressing. You'll need to leave this on for a few days. It may leak and need to be changed. A bruise may develop. After the bone marrow is removed, there is a processing period that may take a few hours. During this time, I encourage you to eat. When you return, the treatment session may last an hour or so. During the treatment part of the appointment, the number of injections is reduced. I direct the injections to the most injured areas and into the joint. I may use fat to place into tears during this treatment process, too. The way that fat is obtained is described below. I will provide nitrous oxide (laughing gas) during this treatment process for nearly everyone. Laughing gas allows for you to deal with the discomfort of the injections, which burn more when they are injected into the soft tissue. If only the joint is injected, there will be little discomfort. Usually only one treatment with stem cells is needed, as most of the pretreatment is done with PRP.

In some people, fat is taken from their midsection or their glute (bum) area. Fat is an insulator and gives the surface of your body contour; it is located between the muscle and the skin. It is a safe way to get your own tissue to use as scaffolding or a graft when there is a tear or hole in the tissue that we want to patch up. When taking fat, I numb the area. Anesthesia combined with saline water (IV solution) is injected in a fan-like arch from this single area. As we wait for this to help break down the fat so that it is easier to extract, we may do the bone marrow stem cell procedure. This order is simply to use the time more efficiently. Once the area is really numb, I will use a long instrument with a number of holes on the side and attach it to a syringe. Pulling back on the syringe generates a negative pressure used to suck up the fat. The goal is to collect around 30 cc of fat from both donation sites on either side of the body. Most people experience pressure while having this done. It is not painful. After the treatment, I will place a compressive dressing over the area. Swelling and bruising may occur.

In review, the day of treatment requires very little preparation if you are being treated with prolotherapy. However, both PRP and stem cell treatments require that you drink half your body weight in water before you come in, as I've mentioned, and they require that you fast for four to five hours beforehand while avoiding fat for twelve hours. The other recommendations, such as medications to avoid and supplements to take, are important to do at this time, as is using a brace or an orthotic. I hope that you are already making some of the changes that were discussed in Chapter 7 to further augment healing. Congratulations on your first treatment! Although there are some variations between treatments, this decision to pursue treatment will reward you after the second or third prolotherapy session and the second PRP session, as you will start to see the benefits.

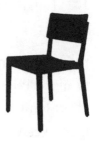

Chapter 9

WHAT CAN I EXPECT AFTER THE TREATMENT?

You are amazing, and your body can heal! Give these positive affirmations to yourself regularly over the next few months. In this chapter, I will discuss what to expect after treatment, but before I do, I want to review the few complications that can occur.

Bleeding and infection are the two most common issues after any treatment that involves needles. In both cases, please call my office or cell phone so we can determine the next course of action. Bruising after a procedure is not unexpected. Some people will tell me that they bruise easily, and bruising would be expected then. Bleeding is more of a concern when an artery is punctured or a vein puncture occurs that doesn't patch itself in the normal amount of time and pressure. Sometimes this occurs after the blood draw to make PRP. With the use of ultrasound, I make an effort to avoid blood vessels. Nerves run right next to blood vessels, and I want to avoid these too. However, if bleeding does occur, I like to be informed. Pressure needs to be placed on the area to stop the bleeding. I don't want a pocket of blood to accumulate in an area. This is known as a hematoma.

Infection is the second most common issue that I am concerned about. This does not usually develop right away. It may be days later. If an infection develops in a joint, this requires an orthopedic surgeon's expertise. This is a big deal. You need to call me, and if I am not available and your joint is red, hot, and swollen, you need to go to the emergency room immediately. We take precautions to prevent this from occurring by making sure that the skin is cleaned with soap, the soap is removed with alcohol, and nothing else is injected or pushed through the skin into the joint. The most common bacteria that causes joint infections lives on the skin. It is for this reason that I don't perform any injections close to an area that is infected or inflamed. However, if a skin infection occurs, this is a different matter. It can be treated with antibiotics.

People's experiences after a procedure vary tremendously. Most people will have a bruised sensation or a deep ache immediately after these treatments. The area feels swollen and motion is restricted. Stiffness is common and may last for a few days. Sharp pain is not one of the normal sensations that people experience. There are many people, especially those who have pelvic, low back, or sacral issues, who experience less discomfort immediately after prolotherapy when trigger points are released. If a nerve is released or a scar is treated, the pain from these structures is reduced immediately. The area may be numb for the first two or three hours depending on the anesthesia that is used and how fast a person breaks it down. This initial discomfort usually last twenty-four to forty-eight hours. However, there are people who experience discomfort for five to seven days. Initially, you can use ice very sparingly for no more than fifteen minutes for people who have a lot of pain. Ice slows down the inflammatory process that is causing the pain. We want the inflammation because that is how healing occurs.

Medications can be prescribed to assist with this but aren't necessary for everyone and may only be needed for the first night. It is really important not to use the anti-inflammatory medications (NSAIDS) like ibuprofen, Advil, Motrin, Aleve, or any that are prescribed by a doctor, such as Celebrex. These medications block inflammation, as described before. The whole purpose of these procedures is to create a localized injury to get your body to assist with healing by allowing it to go through an inflammatory response, which occurs in three phases. The first phase occurs in the first two weeks, the second phase occurs at six weeks to two months, and the third phase occurs around six months. These phases may vary slightly in each individual. Instead of these medications, there are alternative options. If you use these medications to assist with cramping during your periods, homeopathy is a great option. Other safe options include Tylenol or acetaminophen. Herbal or other supplements, such as arnica, Traumeel, turmeric, or curcumin are also fine. There is variation among doctors who do prolotherapy, PRP, and stem cells about whether it's unwise to use even these other supplements described above immediately after the procedure. I am in the camp that the inflammation that is helped by these supplements works on the body differently than the inflammatory cascade that is responsible for healing. However, if you are at all concerned, hold these supplements for three days before and five days after. There are people who use CBD oil as well. Surprisingly heat, especially after the first day, is helpful. Because there can be a lot of injections to an area, the recommendation is that baths and swimming should be avoided for the first twenty-four hours to prevent infection or irritation to the area from chemicals that might resemble infection. Compression of the area that was treated with ACE wraps, Coban wraps, or a neoprene sleeve is also helpful. This helps the area feel more supported.

In all these treatments, massage three days after treatment is okay. Acupuncture is fine. Osteopathic and chiropractic treatments to the soft tissue are fine. High-velocity, low-amplitude (HVLA) manipulation by an osteopath or chiropractor is stressful to the ligaments that were injected and is therefore not recommended. This includes any manipulation that causes a pop. Drop tables should be avoided in pelvic and lower back treatment. Sometimes the original injury was caused by osteopathic or chiropractic treatment. This isn't to say that I don't believe in what they do, it is only to reiterate the skill of the person, the direction of the force, and the amount of force needed to generate a small amount of movement needs to be adjusted for each individual and what their injury is. Some doctors are better at this than others. If you need to be adjusted frequently because you fall out of place, it suggests that your ligaments are not holding you. You are a prime candidate for prolotherapy or PRP if they are extremely loose. In this situation, we will have to talk to whoever is giving you the treatment to find out if they can put you back into place gently while you are getting the treatment.

After the third prolotherapy treatment or the second PRP treatment, I will recommend physical therapy with some very specific limitations. This is true for any area treated because you *can* be injured during physical therapy. The goal during physical therapy is to get your postural muscles, the stabilizing muscles of each joint, to fire or contract at the right time and in the right order. There was a study done on Olympic athletes that had pain. A huge number of these amazing athletes had pain all the time. The pain was not in the muscles that allowed them to move, but in the stabilizing muscle that helped control the motion at the joints. These muscles can be inhibited by pain. These muscles are the ones that I am most interested in rehabbing. I want to improve the biomechanics or the functioning of the area that was injured or led to the injury to prevent further injury. As this occurs, we want to make sure that you have full range of motion and that the motion is controlled both as the muscles are contracting and as they are lengthening under tension. This lengthening is called eccentric control. Many injuries occur as the muscle is lengthening. I also will want to improve your balance on unstable surfaces, such as Swiss Balls or BOSUs. This is important for walking across grassy lawns or on the beach or hiking. The surface in the real world is not flat. Teaching your body to respond to irregularities is part of the rehab.

Body weight exercises are done a few weeks down the line. I had a gymnastics coach who used to say,

"It's not practice makes perfect; it is perfect practice makes perfect." That has stuck with me and applies to this period of time that you are rehabbing. Your head position, your back position, and your shoulder position all have an effect on your posture all the way down to your feet. Likewise, your foot position can have an effect all the way to your head. We want to correct the bad habits that might have led to the injury in the first place before we add strength-based exercises. You might not be able to correct all your postural bad habits in six weeks; instead, this might be a lifelong endeavor. After rehab, the next step might be an appropriate yoga, Pilates, or gyrotonics class. A personal coach who can modify and adjust the exercises to accommodate you as you progress forward is worth their weight in gold. Although I like the concept of CrossFit, I have seen many injuries that have occurred due to people participating in this. Your ability to exercise may vary from day to day depending on your sleep, your stress, the temperature, or what you have done the day before. Please don't expect that your body will perform exactly like it did two days before. Adjust the intensity or duration of your exercise, allowing it to heal between extreme workouts once you get up and moving again. If you have pain, stop. Seek treatment early. It's much easier to treat someone early on in the injury than allowing it to progress.

A flare occurs anywhere from one week to three weeks after treatment with any of these therapies. If the joint is the only thing that is injected, a flare does not occur in the same way. Treatment of the ligamentous or tendon structures that attach to bone are involved with the flare. It is a sign of healing. It usually reproduces what you experienced immediately after the treatment: soreness, a deep ache, or a bruised feeling. If you don't experience it, don't worry; you are probably still healing. The flare catches people off guard. They get a recurrence of pain or discomfort without a warning and without an increase in activity. I tell people to make a mark on their calendar for two weeks after the treatment to avoid the anxiety that occurs when your pain increases. The flare should go away within a couple of days, fading slowly each day. Usually heat is helpful. The recommendations do not change unless there is concern for infection. Fevers, a warm or hot joint, swelling, or a rash need to be evaluated sooner rather than later. Send me a photo by text or email. Call me and be proactive. Don't worry about bothering me. It's important if it is an infection to get treatment immediately.

In general, the more full-body inflammation, the more discomfort after. This includes people with diabetes and anyone with autoimmune issues. The people that I worry about most have gluten, dairy, or other sensitivities and have to avoid foods to keep themselves feeling good. The flare that occurs for weeks after, suggests that these people are not metabolically healthy. This needs to be addressed before any further treatments are done.

Sometimes, people's discomfort starts to worsen again three weeks after the treatment. This is not uncommon. It just means it is time to treat again. By the third prolotherapy treatment, the discomfort or return of the initial symptoms is not as severe as the initial discomfort. It becomes easier to roll over in bed or sit or bend over or reach or hold or lift. The benefits with prolotherapy are subtle. I like to go back to my initial evaluation to review the changes if a patient doesn't recall them, which is common. With PRP, the benefit is often weeks to months down the line. The reason why we treat a few times is to have a compounding amount of healing occurring. I found that I had a residual soreness for months after the stem cell treatment. My function improved first, and the discomfort lagged. The MRI and ultrasound changes lag behind the benefit, meaning you can't see the benefit of healing with these studies. If there are boney changes on x-ray, such as spurs, these will still be present and should not be a way to judge if your treatment was beneficial. A year later, I realized that I didn't have an issue in the same place. Healing occurs over time. The interesting thing that occurs with treatment is that it uncovers underlying issues. Like the onion metaphor, treatment of the outer layer removes that layer as a pain source. As that is healing, the next layer may start to talk. This may be somewhere totally different, or it may be in the same vicinity. I like to treat each of these layers as they show up. Once people realize that I'm treating many areas at the same time, they will come in with an "x" marking where they experience discomfort, pain, or an ache. I love it when they give me a road map. I can see muscle patterns, nerve patterns, and even more importantly fascial patterns. There can be normal patterns or, more likely in these situations, abnormal or compensatory patterns. These areas all need to be treated. Prolotherapy allows for many different areas to be treated at the same time.

It's not uncommon when I am treating women with sacral or pelvic issues that they open up and start to talk about issues with incontinence or how their sex drive has changed or how they have pain with intercourse. The wonderful thing about my training is that I used to deliver babies and do pap and pelvic exams. The combination of those skills and my experience with using platelet-rich plasma has opened up a way to treat these women's health issues. The vaginal area can be injured with vaginal deliveries. It gets stretched during the delivery process. Sometimes everything reverts back to normal, but according to statistics, sixty percent of women over the age of fifty have incontinence issues, meaning coughing, sneezing, lifting, or jumping can result in a loss of urine. This sucks, especially when the kids are growing up and you are ready to do more. Limiting or altering your activity or purchasing pads when you've stopped menstruating is not the end goal. There are surgical options with irreversible risks. Treatment in the vaginal area with platelet-rich plasma is safe. There are no reported long-term side effects from PRP anywhere in studies. There are studies that have shown it to be beneficial. For some women, the benefit is immediate; for some, it takes a few weeks. For some women, it may take one treatment; for others, it may take a few. Sometimes treatment needs to occur the following year. Other times, it may be done sooner or a few years down the line. We are not sure exactly what makes the difference, although hormone replacement improves the benefit of the treatment faster. Any of the recommendations described in the previous chapters will also be beneficial.

In the vaginal area, the numbness from the topical anesthesia may be a few hours. You won't be able to tell when you are urinating. It's a pretty weird sensation. The areas that I treat will have a bruised-like sensation that last a day. Intercourse may be resumed a few days later, but I have known patients to have improved sexual relations that same night. Typically, two areas are injected. However, in patients with pelvic pain or vaginal trigger points, tears, or episiotomy, C-Section scars, or lichen sclerosis, I will treat all these areas as well. Sometimes both the inside of the pelvic bone where the support muscles attach to and the underside of the sacrum need to be treated. In general, after treatment, pelvic rehab is needed. This is much more involved than Kegel exercises. Like any other area of the body, the pelvic floor muscles may have developed bad habits and need to be retrained by physical therapists trained specifically to do this.

There are a few emergent issues that can occur and need to be addressed immediately. These are reasons to call my cell phone or to go to the emergency room. This is not an issue when treating the sacral area, however it may be a rare possibility when treatment of the sacral area is extended up the spine into the rib area. Although ultrasound reduces the chance of this occurring, because the tip of the needle is always visualized, there is a chance with rib and chest treatments that a puncture of the lung can occur. When this occurs, the chest heaviness, or difficulty breathing, is not noticed until a few hours later. This is a situation where it is important to go to an emergency room, not an urgent care. Sometimes the leak is small and is managed by observation. Other times, the leak is larger and can cause the lung to collapse. This requires a chest tube and a hospital stay. I tell people that the risk involved in this happening while using ultrasound is much less than getting in your car to drive each day. However, it is a real risk and needs to be discussed prior to injecting ribs or vertebrae near the lung.

The other big issue that can occur after a treatment is a spinal headache. This occurs most often if epidurals or other more invasive treatment of the spine are done. I don't do these in my office, but it potentially can occur, so I like to let people know that if they have a spinal headache, which is bad headache that is relieved with laying down, it can be treated with the help of another physician. I like to know if this occurs so that I can facilitate getting help for you.

Healing occurs in the same amount of time no matter what treatment you pursue, surgery or injections, with the regenerative orthopedic medicine approach. However, it's possible to cause more inflammation or to treat more areas depending on what regenerative orthopedic treatment is chosen. Prolotherapy treatment allows for a wider and more extensive treatment and for this reason is done initially. Platelet-rich plasma can cause more of an inflammatory response. Stem cells derived from bone marrow improve healing in more difficult areas. The response after treatment can vary between individuals, discomfort lasting one to seven days and the benefit occurring after about two months. A flare is a sign of healing and occurs around two weeks. Exercise limitations during healing are necessary to prevent injury. Physical therapy can be instrumental in retraining muscles to contract at the right time and in the right sequence. Stabilizing muscles or core muscles need to be functional to prevent further injury. Attention to proper posture and movement may be a lifelong process to correct. The goal would be to return you to a life without discomfort or pain where movement is a daily event over the course of six months to a year.

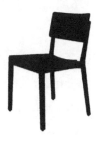

Chapter 10

I AM READY COMMIT TO THE TREATMENT SO THAT I CAN SIT AGAIN

y hope is that, as an educated consumer, as you consider treatment for your pain or injury you recognize that there is value in some things, such as time and experience, which are not reimbursable by any insurance company! You will want to be treated by a physician trained by the conventional medical system and in orthopedic regenerative medicine, who can work in conjunction with your other physicians. Their eight years or more of education has exposed them to inpatient and outpatient treatment.

Most of what I saw as a family doctor was relatively healthy people with issues that cropped up and could be treated at home. Inpatient treatment is what we call hospitals. Because I was trained to the full spectrum of medicine and worked rurally for a few years, I also treated sick patients in the hospital, in the ICU, and after surgery. The first thing that I had to learn was who was sick and how sick they were—whether they were not so sick that they could go home or so sick that they had to go to the hospital. These are important concepts that also apply to injuries and pain. There are areas of the body that require more skill, the spine for example. I treat the spine all the time, to a certain degree. If I am concerned about something that requires equipment or expertise that I don't have, I will tell you and refer you to someone that does. Knowing what you can do and what you shouldn't do is part of our training in medicine.

It is important to recognize that there can be other causes of pain and to evaluate them with a physical exam, laboratory testing, x-rays, MRI, and ultrasound to correlate them to what the patient is experiencing. This can't be done well in fifteen minutes. I'm sure that you expect that this is done completely whenever you approach a medical provider for help. I've given you the information that you'll need to evaluate this for yourself when you are at a doctor's office (refer to Chapter 5). I encourage you to look at the credentials of who is evaluating you and who is treating you. They should be the same person. Specifically, chiropractors and nurses should not be offering you the regenerative orthopedic treatments that I have discussed. This is outside their training.

Anyone can stick a needle into you. That's easy. Not everyone can put the needle in the right spot. Not everyone can treat all the structures surrounding the joint and compose a comprehensive plan from their physical evaluation, laboratory, and radiographic findings. The use of ultrasound is an important aspect of both diagnosis and treatment. All aspects of the treatment should be FDA-approved. This offers protection for you in terms of reducing the chance of infection.

The discussion after you have been evaluated should include the things that you can do to improve your outcome, nutrition, and healthy habits. It should include a discussion about braces, physical therapy, modifications to your exercise routine, supplements, other laboratory testing, and other radiographic studies. Sometimes a referral will be given to another doctor. It is important to share information from the doctors that you have already seen to understand what has been evaluated and the conclusions or recommendations that these other physicians or practitioners have given. The goal is to create a team that communicates well. A well-trained physician, a comprehensive diagnosis, a complete treatment, and an investment from you in your own care will assist you in achieving your goals of stellar health, reduced pain, and improved function.

When you have pain that limits you, the desire to do something different is always on your mind. It is common to have limitations. I call these barriers to making decisions. Sometimes it is fear that prevents us from making optimal decisions. Sometimes it is easier to just avoid the issue. Sometimes there are financial or work or family circumstances that get in the way of planning. Sometimes our ability to think clearly is jaded by the lack of sleep, the fatigue, and the resultant diet from the pain. Sometimes the decision is made without understanding the risks or because the risks are too great or not desirable. Any and all of these issues that are barriers to making decisions are absolutely understandable. The timing of treatment is really important. However, excuses to not make a decision and to invest in your health will ultimately impact your health more negatively.

For me, I recognize that there is a process through which people make decisions. I try to understand your process when you come in for the first visit. I include a personality test with each intake form. Some people have to do a lot of research to come to any decision-making process; others don't like change or need to be in charge or need to talk before they make decisions. Some people like other people to tell them what to do. That is one thing that I will not do. I don't tell you what to do. I offer options for treatment as suggestions. I will discuss all your options for treatment, even surgery; it is an option that you might pursue. If this is the case, I will give you my opinion about the order in which to pursue both surgical and non-surgical treatment. Anything that I do will improve your outcome in the long run. Any of the treatments that I offer have risks but will not permanently alter your anatomy to the point that it creates another issue down the line. For instance, there are no incisional scars, which can cut sensory nerves and become a pain source once they start to heal. I can refer you to studies that you can read if you need help in guiding your decisions. I will answer your questions along the way. I want you to be an informed consumer. I don't want to contribute to your injury by not divulging what to expect during and after the treatment session.

This is your body. You need to know and understand the concepts behind why I am treating it and the expectations during and after the treatment session. I don't want you to walk out of my office with the thought that what I provided you didn't work. The treatments options that I use do work, but it is important to make sure that you are aware of what can be done and what can't be done. Specifically, because so many joint replacements are done each year, it is normal to assume that this is your only treatment option. It is not. Sometimes I offer treatment to help strengthen or stabilize the ligaments and other tissues that are supporting the joint to improve the success of the joint replacement. Some of the joint replacements of the knee, for example, are ligament sparing, meaning your ligaments are left in place to continue to offer support to the joint. If these ligaments are not strong or are injured, the success of the knee replacement is less likely. Other times, after a surgery is done and does not address the pain or there is more discomfort after, I am left with fewer options to work with. This doesn't mean that I can't reduce your discomfort or improve your function. The goals of treatment and the expectations of treatment are different than if I started treating a knee or shoulder, hip, elbow, wrist, thumb, ankle, back, or pelvis prior to arthritis when you first started to experience discomfort. I want you to be a proactive, informed decision maker, to ask questions and get your concerns answered so that you can have the proper expectations during and after the procedure.

None of these options, nor any other option that is available, cures disease or arthritis. The FDA is clear that we are not allowed to say this. However, we can get tendons and ligaments to heal. We have MRI evidence that the cartilage can get thicker with treatment. We know that there are things that can be done to reduce pain. We just can't tell you with certainty for whom this will occur yet. This is true about all aspects of medicine. This is why medicine is an art. Slowly we are figuring out ways to tailor the treatment depending on markers. I am sure that this will be the next wave of the future. What is important is that the sooner you treat, the easier it is to treat and the better the outcome. The longer you wait to address your pain, the harder and longer it can take to heal. This isn't to say that we don't do touch ups years or months later because, in all reality, the goal is to get you moving again, and with that, you could still slip on ice or injure the area again.

I know that in general, your body is amazing! We have an amazing ability to fix things that go wrong. Our DNA is consistently being fixed. As we age, however, it takes much longer to recover from an injury. For instance, when I delivered babies, I had teenage girls deliver their babies, return to their original body weight, and get pregnant again within a few years. They popped out babies with such ease. At thirty-eight, the toll on my body was much longer. In fact, twelve years later, I'm still recovering. My muscle strength has not been the same since. At thirty-five years old, I was riding my bicycle daily. I rode over 4,000 miles that year and was strong. Everything changed during the year that I was pregnant, and without the help of a partner in the house, I didn't recover fast. Hormones play a role in keeping the musculoskeletal system (muscles, tendons, ligaments, nerves, fascia, and joints) healthy. They help orchestrate the behind-the-scenes jobs that promote healing. Having your hormones evaluated and replaced may be a way that you can get your body to start to repair and encourage healing.

I've mentioned other things like restful sleep, nutritious food, plenty of water, and exercise or movement each day as important things that you can do to heal. Changing the habits that cause you to move imperfectly through physical therapy can prevent the injury from recurring. The concept here is that how you live your life and the effort you make to improve the things that you can, one tiny step at a time, have a profound impact on your ability to heal and prevent injury later. If you are invested in your own health, you will feel better. Seeking to make informed decisions about food, for instance, can be time-consuming and overwhelming. Make small, imperfect steps along the way. They are additive. There is always going to be more to learn and differences in opinion and resistance from the kids or the hubby when you make food changes. I get it. It's difficult to figure out ways to augment a meat-and-potato guy's diet when he balks at the sight of vegetables. Changes like avoiding nitrates in meat or buying organic meats or using herbs and spices can be ways to improve their diets, with the addition of supplements.

Talk to me about your concerns; I can usually give some advice or refer you to a website or a colleague who knows more about these things if I can't answer them completely. If you are invested in your health and willing to make changes to improve things, I am your biggest cheerleader.

The thing about pain is that it gets into your head, literally and figuratively. It can also affect the many microorganisms that live in your intestines. These little guys, like it or not, are imbedded into your DNA. As humans, we have only about 26,000 different genes that are unique to humans. The rest of our genes are from microorganisms, bacteria, viruses, fungi, or yeast whose function is to keep us alive or are alive to keep us functioning. The health of these little guys is important. They feel the impact of our own emotional well-being. I believe, for instance, that the types of microorganisms vary between someone who has anxiety versus someone who is calm and centered. There is a role for retraining the relationship you have with pain with your thoughts, which can be done with counseling. I suspect that these microorganisms play a part with the nervous system, as there is a gut-brain interrelationship. Depression or depressive symptoms, such as apathy, sleep issues, hunger issues with weight changes, irritability, hopelessness, sadness, fatigue, mood swings, and concentration issues that can create social isolation or thoughts of suicide are common when pain is present, especially if it is above the level of a five out of ten. It's important to recognize these issues and get support as you are being treated. As you improve, I want to make sure that you have great compensatory habits that prevent you from defining yourself as someone with pain.

It is possible to seek no treatment and be joyful, grateful, and have a purpose in life. I have had these patients in my office. They have figured out ways to alter their brain chemistry or whatever pathway that helps them live with chronic pain and still be positive people. There are therapists that can help you with this. Some people get to this point with the power of prayer or mediation. Usually these people find value in their lives by helping other people. They extend themselves. I can't always fix what caused them this much discomfort, but I can help with giving them time without pain. Sometimes I am able to drop their pain down a few notches completely. The point here is that how you see yourself is as important as anything that I do. If you have been abused or emotionally or physically scarred, the process of working through this to find hope, love, and joy in your life may be how you get out of pain. Remember physical, spiritual, and emotional pain all are felt in the same part of the brain. Please invest in yourself by getting these other issues treated. You are not a victim. You are an undiscovered gem, waiting to radiate!

Injuries untreated become more of burden in the future in many ways: financially, socially, economically, spiritually, and emotionally. I've discussed all of these except the financial ramifications of being in pain. Pain can interfere with your ability to work. This is easy to infer. However, the cost of not being treated or getting the wrong treatment starts to become exponential. Let's say you have pursued a back fusion. We know from research that long-term the areas that are not fused will start to break down. So, one surgery can beget another surgery and possibly more discomfort and less mobility over time. However, if you had your back treated when you first started to get discomfort in your twenties or thirties and corrected your posture, participated in aerobic conditioning, lengthened your tissue through yoga or stretching, and incorporated some strength training, likely this surgery would not have been necessary. This would be a different story if the disc injury occurred in a single event. And even so, it may not be the full cause of your pain.

The point here is that the financial costs are additive over time. Insurance questions always arise when patients are looking into options for treatment. What is covered by the conventional medical system—steroids and many surgeries—can cause and accelerate cartilage damage in the joint. The co-pay or deductible for any surgery will be more than any treatment that I offer. The time off work will be much more with any surgical intervention than what I offer. Insurances don't cover orthopedic regenerative medicine procedures. In this day and age, because insurance is mandated, many people feel entitled to be provided with great healthcare. I have long lost this hope. There were days that I saw sixty patients in a day. In the insurance model, the thing that is valued least is your time with patients. This time to talk, to dive deep into what is troubling someone, to find innovative ways to treat them that are thoughtful, intuitive, comprehensive, and cost effective is not valued in this model. So, I left the model. I am still bothered by Patient X or Patient Z whom I could not effectively help because of the time limitations. What I can promise is more time and dedication to provide you with comprehensive treatment. I'm never going to be a mill. I don't want to be burnt out, depressed, and frustrated again.

I love a challenge or a puzzle. In the past, patients would be referred to me after they had surgery or other procedures that were covered by insurances. Many times, their original issue was still not solved, and they had surgical scars, metal implants, and other limitations that challenged me. It was a practice that was skewed by the population that sought treatment,

I admit. However, with the opioid crisis, I was getting people off of their reliance on pain medications, not adding to it. It is still a process to be treated and to heal from this treatment. It's strange to be the one that colleagues will send someone to when there are no more options. I love working with the people who have had "everything done already" and still experience pain. I love the challenge of solving a puzzle that no one else has solved. But I can't do it without you being invested in your health. This means there is a financial investment too.

Most of my patients with whom I had a long-term relationship will tell you that they felt cared for when they came in to see me. I believe that they felt that I addressed not only their physical needs but also their emotional needs and had conversations that were honest and truthful. I can't promise you the sun and deliver. I *can* give you options that have worked for others. I know what normal healing is and what is not normal. If I don't know something, I have an extensive group of colleagues that I can ask for help. Sometimes two brains are better than one. I expect that you will communicate with me along the way and let me know what you are experiencing. There are new options for treatment that continue to be developed. Some of these options may be more expensive and more precise. As with anything new, I am curious, but I am also careful about safety and long-term side effects that could neg-atively affect my patients. I've been this way all my practicing life. I live by the motto, "First, do no harm."

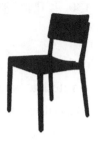

ACKNOWLEDGMENTS

I went back to training after eight years as a family physician, burnt out from the hospital and the clinic work, where I did not feel appreciated or valued. The year of my sports medicine fellowship, I was introduced to many colleagues that I have continued to have relationships with. I am grateful for my friendships with Dr. Paul Johnson, DO of Portland, OR and Dr. Michael Bertram. MD of southern OH/northern KT who are skilled, intelligent, and motivated learning companions. I met them through the Hackett, Hemwell, Patterson Foundation who accepted me for a two-week, hands-on training prolotherapy conference in Honduras. As my late friend Ben Bullington said, "This was the only group of doctors that I wanted to belong to." For me, this continues to hold true, although I've expanded it to other regenerative orthopedics colleagues. This group of physicians wanted to share what they had learned and support each other through the process of continuing to learn. There were egos, no doubt, but the goal was simple: to teach prolotherapy comprehensively and safely to as many physicians who wanted to learn. I continue to honor the HHP Foundation's mission by encouraging new physicians to pursue regenerative medicine and to attend the Wisconsin annual meeting in the fall and to go to Honduras to learn how to treat patients while being supervised. Mary Doherty continues to work for this mission, maintaining Dr. Jeff Patterson, DO's legacy. She is a heart-felt friend. I am thankful for this initial indoctrination into regenerative medicine. She met me at my first AAOM meeting in Washington, DC, in 2006. Since the birth of my child, this has been my favorite conference to attend. It is a reunion of many of the colleagues that I have met along the way that have regenerative medicine practices all over this country and the world. We all continue to grow through experience with patients at different rates. Novel techniques and innovative ways to evaluate areas with ultrasound are shared in the hallways, over meals, and throughout the days. It's a conference where we interact with one another with the goal of sharing. I am grateful for the AAOM as it evolves. I love being around like-minded physicians, who are interested in thoughtfully evolving options for healing musculoskeletal injuries.

This book would not have been possible without the Author Incubator, which provided me with an opportunity to get a book written in twelve weeks during the months that I first opened my doors in Camas, WA after moving my practice from Portsmouth, NH. The beauty of this time was that it solidified what I wanted for and from my practice.

Thank you to David Hancock and the Morgan James Publishing team for helping me bring this book to print.

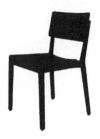

THANK YOU!

Thank you for reading this book! I so hope it was helpful. Welcome to the world of regenerative orthopedic medicine, where pain relief is a goal that occurs without a defined protocol, but rather an individualized or personalized process that is based on a comprehensive evaluation and detailed treatment.

If you are interested in additional information, type **https://vimeo.com/338061476** into your browser to get a free thirty-minute webinar.

I look forward to hearing from you!

https://drstebbing.com
Dr. Jennifer Stebbing, DO
Musculoskeletal & Sports Medicine
info@drstebbing.com
360-258-1746

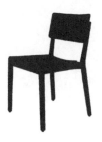

ABOUT THE AUTHOR

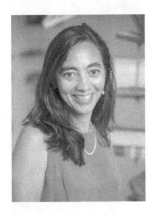

A physician trained in regenerative medicine, Dr. Jennifer Stebbing, DO, wrote *I Can Sit Again: Non-Surgical Treatment for Tailbone Pain* as a guide to help patients who have injured themselves navigate through the complex medical system to find non-surgical solutions to their pain. She is a puzzle master, intuitive listener, and beacon of hope for those who have done "everything" and still aren't fully functional. She heralds from Camas in southern Washington, where she has a physical and telemedical practice.